beat fatigue with yoga

A simple step-by-step way to restore energy

Fiona Agombar

acknowledgements

Firstly I would like to thank Iain McNay and Alex Howard for helping this book to be published again. A huge thank you to Tim Francis, the Patanjali student - for all his help, support and advice. Tim, you are wonderful. Thanks also to Grace Cheetham, my editor when this book was first published.

Thank you to Tanya Roche, a talented photographer, who gave so much of her time during the photographic shoot, even though she is recovering from ME herself. Tanya was in New York on September 11th 2001 staying in an apartment overlooking the World Trade Centre. She witnessed the second aircraft going into the twin towers and the aftermath. As a photographer, her instinct was to grab her camera and she took many reels of film. However, Tanya was then so traumatised by what she had seen that she later destroyed any film that showed images of people involved in this holocaust. She then suffered from Chronic Fatigue Syndrome, partly as a result of the distress of having witnessed 9/11. She came to my yoga class in West London in 2005 and has made huge progress towards getting better - so much so that she was thankfully able to pick up her camera again and take the pictures for this book. Thank you Tanya and also thanks to her assistant Rhea Thierstein. Thanks again to Tim for advising me on alignment during the shoot and Alex for persuading me that the book would be OK if I was in the photographs. Alex also had ME and made a spectacular recovery - you can read his story at the end of this book.

Many thanks to my teachers, past and present, who continue to inspire me with my yoga practise: Angela Stevens, Chris Jagger and Bill Feeny. Thank you to Jackie Sievewright, Theresa Coe and Jayne Roscoe for your love and friendship. Thank you also to Martina Dodder whom I met in India and who has widened the possibilities for my yoga teaching; the universe led me to you. I would also particularly like to thank all my students who are my greatest teachers. Finally, I would like to dedicate this book to my mother Hazel with all my love.

Fiona Agombar worked in television and ran her own public relations business before she became ill with M.E. in 1990. She was a Trustee of Action for ME for ten years. She now regularly contributes to *Interaction*, the charity's magazine, as well as other health journals. After she recovered, Fiona started teaching yoga in 1999 and now works extensively in therapeutic yoga. Fiona runs yoga classes in London and retreats all over the world.

First published by Element Books Ltd 1999
This Edition 2016

This edition published 2016 by Cherry Red Books, Power Road Studios,
114 Power Way, London W4 5PY

ISBN: 1 901447 456

Design: Dave Johnson

Preface

Since I wrote the first edition of this book, back in 1997, I have continued to grow and learn through my yoga practice and I sincerely hope that this book can help you. What I would like to emphasise is that yoga is not gymnastics designed for only the very fit who maybe able to get themselves into difficult poses. Yoga is for absolutely anyone - young, old, fit or sick. Yoga is essentially a spiritual practise aimed at quietening the mind to prepare mind and body for meditation. You may not be interested in the spiritual side of yoga but, nevertheless, everyone can benefit from learning to still the mind. Thousands of years ago Patanjali, often called the father of yoga, wrote that yoga is about controlling the thought-waves of the mind. If you can bring peace and calm to your mind and learn to live more in the present moment, rather than allowing thoughts to control you as they dash between the past and the future, then you will have taken the first steps towards not just a healthy body, but a contented mind and spirit. And, you will have lots more energy! Practice regularly and you will reap huge rewards.

Om Shanti,

Fiona Agombar, 2013

Contents

foreword

There are many self-help books on the shelf these days but very few are written from such direct experience of not only the condition but also of the recovery. In this book Fiona shares with the reader her path back to a quality of life that had been denied her by ME, a debilitating disorder of which the most distressing symptom is extreme fatigue.

Fiona soon realised that, through Yoga, she had the means to improve her quality of life – the true foundation for self healing. Yoga led her to understand that she had the tools to overcome her condition, the tools which are so well presented in this book of Yoga.

I see this text not only as a guide back to good health but also as a guide to prevention. The fact that we live in a society dedicated to aggression and gain puts us all under the kind of pressure which few of us are immune to.

The core of Fiona's book is self-realisation, the realisation that however severe the condition there is a path that we can take to recovery. I have no hesitation in recommending this book to you as part of your healing journey.

Bill Feeney
Director, Yoga for Health Foundation

Introduction

You're tired all the time, exhausted even – and you want to know how you can get more energy. Can this book help you? Well, I have witnessed many, many people with fatigue improve their quality of life dramatically by using yoga. With practice, you will become calmer, less stressed and more content. In fact, if you really apply what you learn from this book, you will soon notice a huge improvement in your health and stamina.

Think about this. Wouldn't it be wonderful if you could tap into an endless source of energy? Wouldn't it be wonderful if you had so much vitality that you felt as if you were plugged into a main electrical circuit, rather than having a battery that runs flat all the time? Yoga can help you tap into this energy – the universal energy that is all around us. Quantum physics acknowledges that the universe consists of patterns of energy, of which atoms are a part. What you may not know is that the philosophy of yoga is based on the concept of how to use this energy, which is call prana, a Sanskrit word meaning the first unit of life force, or the energy which sustains life and creation. Prana is said to be the sum total of all the energy that is manifest in the universe. Some say prana is to yoga what electricity is to modern civilization. Vigour, power, vitality, life and spirit are all forms of prana.

This sounds almost too good to be true – can there really be such an energy force that we can discover? In this book we are going to look at prana, and I will show you how you can use this energy and gain endless vitality. There are some simple postures to practise, together with visualizations and breathing exercises that will dramatically increase your stamina – and really help you to beat fatigue. Like a car battery, you need to put yourself on charge to make use of this vital life force. If you can do this, you will have the key to mental and physical health. That is what this book is about – helping you to gain more energy and vitality through the use of special yoga exercises.

what causes **fatigue?** 1

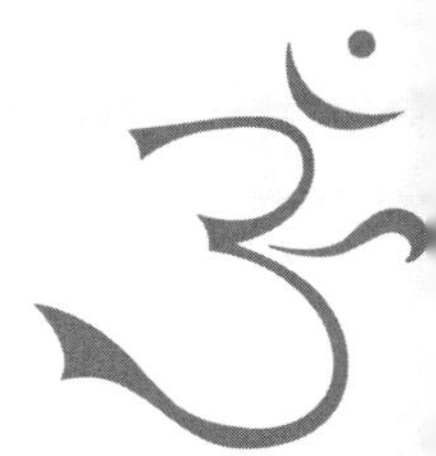

Yoga helps bring balance into your life. The word yoga, meaning 'union', refers to the balance between mind, body and spirit. You can think about balance in your life in terms of how much energy you use up and how much you put back in. Imagine that your stamina is like a bank account. You can't keep taking endlessly from your account. When you use up your energy, you must put something back into the account, such as resting between your daily activities, practising relaxation at least once a day, and eating nutritious food. You need to look after yourself!

One of the main reasons you've bought this book may be because you feel tired for much of the time. But do you know why you feel tired – and how would you define how you feel? Is it that you generally feel 'below par', as if you are unable to function properly? Have you noticed a gradual drop in your energy levels? Do you feel unwell all of the time? Is this your only symptom? Or is your fatigue so severe that it interferes with your everyday life and actually stops you from working, or doing things you usually enjoy? Whatever your symptoms, we will now look at the most common reasons for fatigue.

Everybody feels tired if they over-exert themselves – this is normal. But stress, a poor diet, doing too much and repeated infections on top of a run-down system can cause you to feel an unnatural tiredness. These factors can also lead to blocked chakras. In yoga, chakras are thought of as energy centres through which prana or universal energy is picked up. If they are not functioning properly, you will feel very unwell. I'll explain more about prana and how you can work on your chakras to increase your energy levels in Chapter 3.

Please bear in mind that it is important to discuss your health with your doctor. Fatigue can be a sign that there is something seriously wrong. Cancer, heart disease, HIV, lupus, multiple sclerosis, rheumatoid arthritis, diabetes, an underactive thyroid and lung disease are just a few examples of what can cause serious exhaustion. However, fatigue that seems to have no cause is incredibly common. In his book *Tired all the Time*, Dr Alan Stewart, says that in the US, fatigue accounts for 24 per cent of adults seeing their doctor. A report commissioned in the UK by the Royal Colleges of Physicians, Psychiatrists and General Practitioners in 1996 said: 'Fatigue is one of the most common complaints encountered in community health services.'

Fatigue often arises from the long-term running down of the body's system, so I'm going to start by looking at stress. This is a very common cause of exhaustion - more common, in fact, than most of us realise.

Lifestyle and Stress

Stress can have a profound effect on your health at all levels and is one of the major reasons for fatigue. Strangely enough, you may not even be aware that you are under stress. So you do need to think about this. First of all, ask yourself: am I doing too much in my life? Am I actually taking out more than I am putting back in - in terms of making my own space in my life, having adequate rest and relaxation and proper nutrition? The way in which our bodies deal with pressure and strain - which is called our 'fight or flight' response - is not really equipped to cope with the stresses of modern-day living.

If constantly triggered, this response can cause extreme tiredness. It is triggered by your thoughts; your perception of events. Think about something that makes you very anxious. You may feel your heart start to pound and your hands become clammy. Your mouth may go dry and you may notice butterflies in your stomach - this is because your digestive juices have slowed right down. This can create problems with absorbing the nutrients from your food and is one of the reasons why it is advisable to eat while you are calm and not under stress. So, even how you think about an event affects your stress levels.

Our ancestors needed the 'fight or flight' response in order to deal with physical threats or emergencies - by running away from wild animals, for example. When your body is under stress, the autonomic part of your nervous system cuts in and your body leaps into action. This is largely unconscious - in other words, you have little control over what happens next. The hypothalamus gland in the brain, which monitors your systems, sends electrical and chemical messages to another part of your brain, the pituitary gland, which is largely responsible for hormone production in your body. A hormone called ACTH is then sent to your adrenal glands, which release over 30 chemicals, including cortisol and adrenaline. (You know what this feels like - the speedy, anxious feeling you get from adrenaline!) In addition, glucose is released from your liver into the blood in order to give you a boost of energy; your blood pressure and heart rate rise; your digestive juices slow down or even stop; the muscles of your neck and shoulders tense; you breathe faster and less deeply to take in more oxygen; and you perspire.

This is all very well if you take the appropriate action - like running very fast - but it is not so good in a situation where you don't need this response. If you are arguing with your boss or bank manager, or in a traffic jam, for example, you don't need your blood pressure to rise or your breathing rate to change. The problem gets even worse if your body adapts to this 'fight or flight' response and doesn't relax afterwards - which it won't if you are constantly exposed to what you perceive as stressful situations. Later on I will show you how to control this potentially exhausting situation.

The Three Stages of Stress

The Canadian researcher Hans Selye noticed that the body goes through three stages when it is exposed to stress for a long time.

1 The Alarm Stage

This is the basic 'fight or flight' response as just described. When the body returns to normal, you may feel very tired.

2 The Adaptation Stage

This is the stage at which you should start to take notice, before you pass on to the third, more serious, stage. As you start to get used to being stressed, you may feel below par most of the time because your 'fight or flight' mechanism is constantly switched on. If you are under constant pressure, the problem is that your nervous system is unable to bring the body back to its normal level. The worrying thing is that you may not know that you are stressed and have reached this second stage, because you get used to living life at this pace. This is why it is so important in yoga to learn to listen in to your body, so that you can take the appropriate action.

Some of the clues that you may have reached the Adaptation Stage include a sense of speeding up: talking and eating quite quickly, drinking fast and working at high speed. It's a bit like having your foot always on the accelerator pedal. This Adaptation Stage of stress is very tiring, as you are continually depleting your body of its natural reserves. As you can imagine, you are likely to start to suffer from problems such as digestive disorders, high blood pressure, hyperventilation, anxiety, irritability and depression. You may have additional fatigue caused by low blood sugar as your adrenal glands start to become inefficient and the adrenaline can't maintain your blood sugar level. (Remember, the body is taking glucose from the liver.) Other problems you may notice are that you become more susceptible to illness; you may suffer from mood swings, headaches, heart problems and insomnia. At this point, you will probably start relying on stimulants - like coffee, alcohol, cigarettes and sugary foods, even drugs - to get more energy. This is the worst thing you can do: your body needs better nutrition to support the adrenal glands, not stimulants to put a further burden on them!

3 The Exhaustion Stage

This is the final stage of continual stress, when the body has pushed itself too far and reaches the stage of utter exhaustion or burn-out. This is very serious as it can lead to total collapse, nervous breakdown, heart attack, ulcers, severe depression and anxiety, and severe fatigue. Doctors know the problems stress can create but many of us are not willing to take the steps to do something about it. It is so much easier not to change our lifestyle and just to carry on, ignoring our symptoms.

Ways to Deal with Stress

- First of all, listen to your body and recognise if you are under stress. Once you start to see the familiar signs, such as tense muscles, fast respiration and a racing heartbeat, you can consciously practise relaxing your body and slowing down your breathing. This will bring down your heart rate and control other symptoms of stress. (See the breathing exercises in Chapter 4.)
- Every day, practise a relaxation posture such as the Pose of Complete Rest (see page 82). Try not to think of this as another thing you need to make time for – think of it as your treat.
- Regular practice of yoga poses (see Chapters 5-8) will really help your stress levels.
- Whenever you feel under pressure, make a conscious effort to slow down your breathing and to breathe from your diaphragm (see page 24). Also, be aware of your posture.
- Meditate every day (see Chapter 11).
- Eat a good diet. This is so important that I will refer to it constantly throughout this chapter. I will then explain what a good yoga diet is in more detail in the next chapter. Do remember for now that the more you suffer from stress, the more tempting it is to take short-cuts and to eat ready-prepared meals and junk food. Certain nutrients are required for the 'fight or flight' response, and if you are nutritionally deficient – or under constant stress – you may exhaust your adrenal system even more. Avoid sugar, alcohol, caffeine and stimulants.
- Start to be aware of how you think. Changing how you think will take a lot of practice. If you perceive a situation as negative, or with fear and anger, try to

see the positive side of things. Of course, this is easily said but much more difficult to do. Is the situation teaching you a valuable lesson? Do you perhaps feel trapped, or feel that your life is hopeless and that you are stuck with something you hate – a job, relationship, financial commitment, or whatever? This is seldom true; change is always possible if you have the courage to recognise that you need to take action. Look at your lifestyle and how it is affecting your health. Resolve to make changes that will reduce your stress levels if you can. Meanwhile, if you feel under pressure, thinking calm, healing thoughts is a powerful tool for coping with problems. Whenever something dreadful happens in my life, I remind myself that I have to accept that some things can't be changed and that even pain eventually passes. We all have to learn to let go of the past and move on. Acceptance is not the same as putting up with a situation, but if you are calm, it is easier to see what action you could take to improve it. If you learn to control your emotions, you will be in command of your feelings – not controlled by them. This is not the same as not showing your feelings – if you keep such a tight rein on them that you hide them, this will only increase your stress. Rather, allow your feelings to happen. Try to be present more in the here and now

- Accept what can't be changed, but control what can – as demonstrated by the third canoeist in the following analogy:

There were three canoeists on a rough sea. The first canoeist tried to steer against the sea with all his might. After a few hours, he was completely exhausted and gave up; the sea overwhelmed him and he drowned. The second canoeist didn't bother to fight the sea -he just let his canoe drift wherever the waves wanted to take him. He ended up being dashed onto the rocks. The third canoeist also knew he couldn't fight the sea - but he knew too that it would be foolish and weak just to drift. He used his paddle to steer a course, avoiding the rocks but harnessing the power of the sea to take him in the right direction, towards the safety of the harbour.

In this story, you are the canoeist and the sea is your life. You shouldn't fight and struggle against the things you can't change, but you do need to steer yourself in a positive direction if you want to avoid being overwhelmed with stress and tension.

A Simple Visualisation

Lie down and close your eyes. Think very hard about anything that is making you feel unhappy or stressed. Now try to relax your body as much as you can. Imagine that you are blowing into a large red balloon. You are going to breathe all your stress into this balloon. Each time you breathe out, the balloon gets bigger. It is filling up with all your negative feelings. Anger, fear, hopelessness, grief, despair are all blown into the balloon. As the balloon gets larger, imagine that you are tying it at the neck. Now let it go so that it can start to float away. On each out-breath, it goes further up into the sky, until you can't see it any more. Now, on each in-breath, breathe peace and calm into your body until it fills your whole being with relaxation.

Colin's Story

I am 60 and work as a commercial manager in the construction industry. I have always set myself very high standards of achievement – I am a real perfectionist. My philosophy has always been 'I must try my hardest', which I thought gave me a grip on life and my behaviour. In the last few years, work has been getting more and more hectic. I guess I was suffering from all kinds of problems – a heart murmur, digestive problems, anxiety and fatigue – but I ignored these symptoms as much as I could.

One day, on a particularly long journey, the traffic was atrocious and I decided to stop at a friend's house. This I did, but suddenly my body seemed to take over and I felt completely drained of energy. I slept for four days without a break, and I still found I had no energy. I tried to go back to work, telling myself it was all in my mind, but I found it impossible to concentrate. I was completely physically drained. I couldn't seem to walk more than 30 or 40 yards.

By a series of coincidences, someone recommended that I attend a yoga retreat for a week. I was sceptical at first, but I went along to see what would happen. Practising yoga, meditation and relaxation slowly built up my energy. My body felt in tune with the yoga postures, and every day a light shone brighter. I went home and took another three weeks' rest before I returned to work. During this time, I realised the importance of discipline, and I practised yoga every morning for 40 minutes. Each day I had a period of meditation and relaxation. This all energised me. Now, I practise yoga and meditate every day, and seem to be in complete control of my life. At work, I take a break at lunchtime and have a walk. I try to follow a diet based on the yoga principles. I feel 10 years younger, happy, and at peace with all that surrounds me. My world is full of love for all people and the universe. You may think it sounds like a cliché - but when I found yoga it was a turning point in my life!

Other Conditions Affecting Energy Levels

Allergies and Intolerances

If you are allergic to a food or substance, your immune system will usually respond in such a way that you will have a severe reaction. A true allergy invokes the response of your immune system, usually raising histamine levels. This means that after eating the offending food, or breathing in a chemical or pollen to which you are allergic, you may have a violent reaction - such as a skin rash, streaming eyes or a runny nose. Examples of this kind of allergy include eczema, asthma and coeliac disease (an allergy to gluten). It is becoming increasingly common, however, for people to develop food or environmental sensitivities. As a result of a low-grade chronic immune response, you may experience symptoms you find difficult to define - mood disorders, concentration difficulties, breathing problems, weight fluctuations, erratic heartbeat, skin disorders, joint problems, irritable bowel syndrome - and fatigue.

Allergies and food or chemical intolerances are more common today because our immune systems have to put up with so much more than they did 50 years ago. Pesticides, food additives, antibiotics and pollution are just a few of the things that can challenge and overload your immune system. By this I mean that the defence system of your body is so overworked that it can't cope as effectively, and eventually breaks down. A poor diet can add to this picture. If you are not eating properly, you are not supporting your immune system and helping it to cope.

Stress can also increase the likelihood of your developing allergies or food sensitivities – if you are eating when stressed, your body is not producing enough digestive juices to help with the proper absorption of food. Worse, if you develop candida, you may suffer from leaky-gut syndrome, which means that undigested particles of foods can pass through your gut wall. This may cause your immune system to over-react, because it sees these food particles as foreign bodies – or allergens. Yet again, you can see that diet has a vital contribution to make in beating fatigue.

If you can identify the substances to which you are sensitive and avoid them, this can greatly help your energy levels. This can be difficult, however, because if you continue to eat a substance to which you are intolerant, your body will adapt and the reactions become less severe and more vague. It then becomes difficult to identify the offending food – it is easier to detect when you have a more obvious and severe allergic response. Worse still, you may even crave the foods to which your body is sensitive! This is because you will get a temporary lift as adrenaline is produced to fight the reaction. However, this beneficial effect disappears after a couple of hours and you may then feel unwell again.

The best way to discover if you suffer from food or chemical sensitivities is to go on a modified fast for five days. This gives your body time to rest. You will then be able to 'unmask' culprit foods when you reintroduce them gradually, because if you do have an intolerance, you will have a more severe reaction when you next eat the offending food. This is best done under supervision. However, it will also help if you eat only organic food, use unperfumed products in the house and bathroom, and avoid pollution and sprays wherever possible so that you are then not putting such a load on your immune system.

Anaemia

Anaemia refers to a deficiency in the blood (usually of red blood cells) or low levels of haemoglobin (the red blood pigment that contains iron and carries oxygen around the body). Anaemia is not caused just by an iron deficiency. It may be due to a lack of copper, folic acid or vitamins B12 and C. It is usually a gradual process: your red cell activity moves slowly away from its normal range until you notice that you feel tired and run down. If you are anaemic, check with your doctor and supplement your diet with vitamins C, B12, and folic acid as well as iron. Anaemia is particularly common in women who drink a lot of tea, as the tannin can leech away at your iron supplies. If you are a tea-drinking vegetarian, and suffer from fatigue, do consider taking an iron supplement.

Candida or Gut Dysbiosis

You may have heard about candida as it has received a lot of attention in recent years. If you are suffering from fatigue, candida is certainly something you should consider as a possible cause. Candida albicans is a yeast-like mould which lives in all of us. It lives on the skin and in mucous membranes, such as the digestive tract. Usually, its presence causes no problem as it is kept in check by friendly bacteria. The problem arises only when there are not enough of these friendly bacteria. A number of factors contribute to candida overgrowth:

- antibiotics (which kill off the friendly bacteria)
- the contraceptive pill (which affects hormone function; candida thrives when progesterone is high)
- steroid drugs
- a weakened immune system
- stress
- poor nutrition (such as a diet high in sugar).

The situation is made worse if candida gets a grip on your digestive system and puts down root-like structures. This can cause your gut to leak, allowing partly digested foods to pass into your bloodstream. This can then make you sensitive to certain foods, which may well compound your tiredness. As the candida dies off, it gives off toxins that can make you feel very unwell.

The symptoms of candida or gut dysbiosis include:

- severe fatigue
- headaches
- foggy head
- difficulty in concentrating
- food cravings
- mood swings
- thrush
- itchy anus
- constipation
- diarrhoea
- bloating
- gas.

It may also cause irritable bowel syndrome. You may have some of these symptoms – you are unlikely, or very unlucky, if you have them all. If you suspect that you have candida, do see a practitioner who can test you and give you the appropriate treatment. This will involve following a diet that excludes all forms of sugar, yeast and alcohol, and includes supplements to help kill off the candida and repopulate the gut with friendly bacteria. After this regime, your energy levels should improve dramatically.

Depression

I have already explained that you may not know your fatigue is caused by stress because you adapt to it. Likewise, you may be suffering from depression, which will make you feel very tired, without realizing that depression is causing your exhaustion. This may sound strange, but it is true that sufferers of depression can fail to realise that their mood has gradually lowered, until they find that their world is hopeless and grey.

Depression is caused by a biochemical change in your brain. Your moods are regulated by neurotransmitters, which send messages from one neuron to another. A number of chemicals help your neurotransmitters in different parts of your nervous system, and a normal mood requires a careful balance of these. Depression is usually caused by a deficiency of the neurotransmitters norepinephrine and serotonin. As well as causing a low mood, a lack of these chemicals may also cause fatigue. Drugs that help to relieve depression increase the amounts of these chemicals - but activity such as yoga has been shown to help alleviate moderate depression because it helps to increase endorphins in the brain - your natural 'feel good' chemicals.

To find out if you are depressed, ask yourself the following:

- Does your world seem hopeless and your outlook bleak?
- Do you look forward to anything?
- Do you feel sad, tired and generally uninterested in life?
- Do you find it difficult to relate to those around you?
- Do you wake up early?
- Do you suffer with low self-esteem?
- Do you see yourself as a failure and feel that your life is out of control?
- Do you have unexplained aches and has your appetite changed?

If you have any of the above symptoms, then you could be suffering from depression and you should consider seeing your doctor. Do remember, however, that most of us have times when we feel low or depressed. It is a normal response to many of life's stresses. For example, if you have lost your job, have poor health or someone close to you has died, then depression would be a normal response. It only becomes a problem when it is out of proportion to events and continues past the point that you can cope with in everyday life.

Depression may be caused by how you view the world. Are you happy with what you have? Does your fantasy of life match how your life really is? This is where yoga can help. Yoga teaches us acceptance of how life is; it shows us the illusion of things such as material possessions and teaches us to live more in the present and accept what we have. The root of unhappiness is often caused by not being satisfied with what we have and wanting more. Perhaps you need to lower your expectations and learn to accept what can't be changed.

Depression may also be caused by stress, so if you think you have a problem with low mood, look again at the suggestions given on coping with stress. Meanwhile, try to set small goals for yourself and practise a few yoga postures every day. Nutrition can dramatically affect your mood. Lack of the B-vitamins and amino acids found in protein, for example, can contribute to depression, as can sugar, caffeine and alcohol. Following the diet recommended in Chapter 2 may well help.

Hormone Imbalance

We looked at some of the hormones that affect fatigue when we examined stress - adrenaline and insulin were just two that were mentioned. Your hormones can have a profound effect on your energy levels. If you are a woman and you suffer from premenstrual syndrome (PMS), you will know that this is true! Men are also affected by their hormones.

Your hormone or endocrine system is largely controlled by the pituitary gland in your brain. There are various hormones, the imbalance of which can bring about changes in the body's chemistry, leading to symptoms including mood changes and fatigue. Your hormone balance can be affected by various lifestyle factors such as diet and exercise and getting out of rhythm with your cycles. If you go to bed during the day and not at night, for example, your pituitary gland will eventually stop producing the hormone melatonin at the right time to help you sleep - and this will have a knock-on effect on other hormones.

One hormone worth mentioning here is thyroxine, produced by the thyroid gland. If your thyroid gland is not producing enough thyroxine, your body will be unable to convert your food into energy. Thyroxine stimulates the body's cells to take in more oxygen to help with this conversion. The symptoms of hypothyroidism (an underactive thyroid) include weight gain, undue sensitivity to cold, aches and pains - and fatigue. Your thyroid function can be checked with a simple blood test. There is a current theory that people who suffer from Chronic Fatigue Syndrome (CFS) will often show a test result at the lower end of the normal range – and that they get better with a low dose of thyroxine. By all means check with your doctor if you think having a hormone test will help, but meanwhile practise your yoga postures and eat a balanced diet to help your endocrine system in general.

Hyperventilation

I have already mentioned that you may not be aware you are suffering from certain states, such as stress and depression. The same can be said for hyperventilation, which can also cause profound fatigue. It is very common, but if you are a sufferer it is very unlikely that you will be aware of it. Hyperventilation is defined as breathing at a rate greater than your body needs. People who hyperventilate tend not to use their diaphragm when they breathe, but breathe only from their upper chest area.

When we talk about breathing, it is vital that you understand exactly what your diaphragm is and what it does. The diaphragm is a large sheet of muscle attached to your spine at the back, and to your bottom ribs at the front. When you breathe in, your diaphragm ensures that your lungs are fully inflated. When you breathe out, your diaphragm rises in a cone shape, so that it acts like a piston. When your posture is good and your muscles properly in balance, your diaphragm can help to balance and relax your body. You'll see why this is later when you read the section on posture.

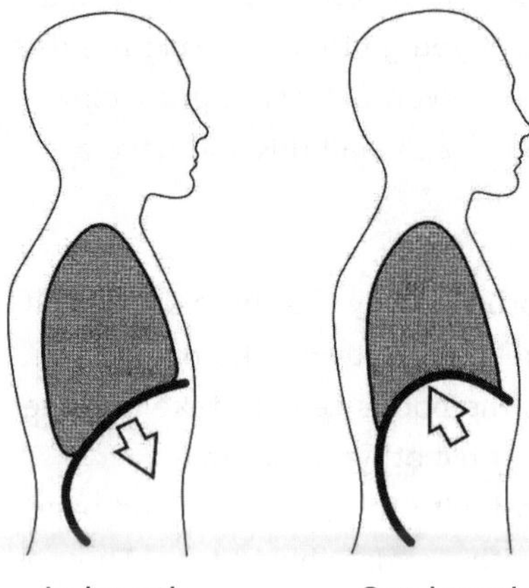

Movement of the diaphragm

Most people think that they need lots of oxygen for energy. What you actually need is a balance of oxygen and carbon dioxide, and if you breathe too fast you breathe off too much carbon dioxide. What then happens is that the pH of the blood gradually becomes too alkaline. This can have a serious effect on your muscles and nerves. Also, if you shallow breathe, your levels of magnesium will be used up, and magnesium deficiency has been shown to be a contributing factor in Chronic Fatigue Syndrome. Symptoms that may indicate you are hyperventilating include talking too fast, vivid dreams, a tingling numbness in your hands, difficulty in getting your breath, yawning and sighing a lot, and difficulty in swallowing. As the problem becomes more severe, you may eventually experience panic attacks, phobic states, and a feeling of being 'spaced out' or unreal.

Hyperventilation may be caused by stress – you will remember that when the 'fight or flight' mechanism kicks in, your breathing rate increases. You will also remember that if you are under constant pressure, this mechanism may not shut down completely, so that you will continue to breathe fast and your body will get used to breathing in this way. Because breathing too rapidly activates adrenaline, you will also find that it makes you very tense, and you may suffer from painful muscles. Food intolerance and allergies can also result from hyperventilation as the lower levels of carbon dioxide release histamine in your body, which may contribute to allergic reactions. Low blood sugar and poor posture can also add to the picture of a rapid breathing pattern.

Your breathing is largely driven by your unconscious, but you can override it and learn to breathe properly. If you are breathing more than 18 times a minute, you are probably breathing too fast. Try to slow down to a cycle of 12 breaths a minute. A cycle is one in-breath and one out-breath. Place your hands on your lower ribs just above the abdomen so that you can feel the movement of your diaphragm as you breathe. Practise this for 10 minutes, twice a day. Remember to breathe through your nose if you can – which will stop you breathing in great gulps of air. In yoga, you should always breathe through your nose anyway, as the fine hairs in your nostrils help to filter out toxins. Although it may be necessary to breathe fast if you are being chased by a wild animal, it is inappropriate in most everyday situations, such as in a traffic jam or during an argument with someone!

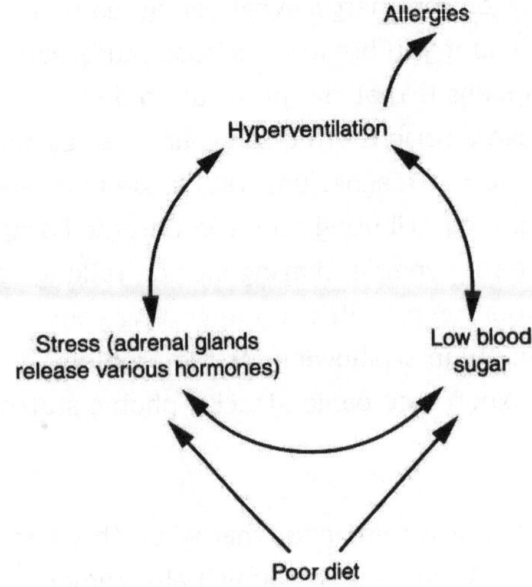

The hyperventilation cycle

Hypoglycaemia

Hypoglycaemia literally means a low level of sugar in the blood. It is a very common cause of fatigue, especially now that some nutritionists are encouraging people to eat lots of carbohydrates and recommending that certain combinations of food - protein and starches, for example - should not be eaten together (food combining). If you don't eat enough protein and complex carbohydrates in combination, however, this can lead to the state of low blood sugar or hypoglycaemia. As with stress, it is very possible to suffer from this condition without realizing it.

We all need glucose for energy, and our body converts the food we eat into glucose so that it can be used for our brain and nervous system. On a reasonable diet, this conversion takes place over a period of several hours from the breakdown of fats, proteins and carbohydrates. Your blood sugar level lies within a certain normal range under these conditions. When you eat, this level rises as you absorb the glucose from your food - then it falls back to normal. The problem starts when your blood sugar level rises too high, too quickly - and this will happen if you eat sweet, sugary food or fast-releasing carbohydrates such as white pasta, cakes or white rice. These foods are converted to glucose much faster than proteins and complex starches, such as brown rice or products made with wholegrain flour. Your pancreas tries to compensate for this steep rise in blood sugar by releasing insulin, which then tries to push your glucose into the body's cells. In this way, glycogen and insulin are competing to stabilise your blood sugar level. But if it has gone too high, the insulin will make it drop – sometimes very low – below the normal range.

If your blood sugar is low, you may experience symptoms such as:

- irritability (especially before a meal)
- nausea
- faintness
- weakness
- dizziness
- lack of concentration
- shakiness
- headaches
- anxiety
- mood swings
- an overwhelming desire to binge.

You will also feel very tired. You are likely to hyperventilate too, which will add to the picture of stress and fatigue. You may have only some of these symptoms but you are most likely to experience them between meals, mid to late morning and mid to late afternoon, for example. You will then crave and eat sugary foods to give you a quick lift. You may crave to the point of addiction – you *have* to have that chocolate bar, glass of wine or jam doughnut! A couple of hours later, you will feel very tired as your blood sugar level drops again. Incidentally, this is why dieters often fail – if they don't eat properly and become hypoglycaemic, they have overwhelming desires to binge so as to raise their low blood sugar level.

To add to this picture, if you have low blood sugar, your body produces more adrenaline, which puts a strain on your adrenal system. This can trigger the 'fight or flight' response, giving you a false feeling of energy and alertness, which in the long run is very tiring. So, indirectly, being hypoglycaemic will add to any stress or tiredness you are experiencing -and vice versa.

The way to break the roller-coaster pattern of high/low blood sugar is very simple. You need to aim to keep your blood sugar level stable. This will take only a few days, during which time you may crave sweet foods - but stick with it, as the results can be remarkable.

- Always eat some form of protein with your starches. So don't have a piece of toast or crispbread on its own, but have something like cottage cheese, tahini or almond butter with it. Don't eat just a jacket potato and salad, but have them with a protein such as pulses or fish. The Hay diet, which recommends keeping protein and starches separate, may work for some people, but if you are hypoglycaemic, it is a bad idea.
- Eat every three to four hours. Good snacks include nuts and seeds.
- Avoid coffee and alcohol - they will make your problem worse.
- Avoid sweets and sugar at all costs. Do not eat food that contains white flour or white rice. Buns, cakes and desserts are out.
- Don't miss meals and always eat a good breakfast that includes some form of protein. Eat foods with a high G.I. index.
- Physical exercise improves blood sugar control, so practise your yoga postures.

Low Blood Pressure

People talk a lot about the problems of high blood pressure. If you have low blood pressure however, this will make you feel dizzy and fatigued. Low blood pressure is actually classed as a medical condition in Germany, although in other countries it is considered normal, even though it can leave you feeling tired and weak. If your blood pressure is low, the inverted yoga postures (such as the Shoulder Stand) described in Chapter 8 will help.

Posture and Energy Levels

Correct posture is so important that I want to explain how it affects your health at all levels. You will then see how the yoga poses will give you more energy as your posture improves. When you are tired, you are more likely to flop or slump in your chair. Unfortunately, this will make you more tired as major organs of your body become restricted. Your heart will beat faster and your rib area will tense so that you can't breathe properly - and this will make your thoughts race. This then becomes a vicious circle - the more fatigued you become, the more you slump, until you are almost curling into yourself, which in turn can make you feel more exhausted and depressed!

The health of your spine is essential for your wellbeing. Not only does it support your body, but it also contains the spinal cord, the main route for information from the nervous system to your brain. The cerebrospinal fluid contained in the spinal cord provides the brain and nerve tissues with oxygen and nutrition, and helps with the drainage of waste products. Amazingly, this fluid has a physical potency of energy with its own rhythm and pulsation - which fluctuates at 10-14 cycles per minute in healthy adults. Fear can actually stop this fluid from flowing! The cerebrospinal fluid is also vulnerable to outside influences such as tea, coffee and stress - and, of course, poor posture.

The cerebrospinal fluid affects the biochemistry of every cell in the body and plays an important role in internal tissue respiration. Any disturbance in the spinal fluid may show in your breathing - and so yoga breathing can help in keeping this fluid healthy. Any osteopath who uses the sacrocranial technique, works with the pulsation of the spinal fluid and its link to the brain. When your cerebrospinal fluid is flowing properly, your energy levels will be enhanced.

Poor posture restricts your digestion. If your colon is compressed, it is difficult for it to function efficiently and you may suffer from all kinds of digestive disorders, including irritable bowel syndrome. If you slump, you also restrict your diaphragm, which can lead to various other problems. If you can't breathe properly, you will probably start to hyperventilate, which in turn can affect your mental outlook and energy levels. (On a visit to a psychiatric hospital, I noticed all the patients had terrible posture – some were slumped very far forward. I wondered if their posture contributed to their condition – or was it the other way around?) Without doubt, if you start to slump forward, you will feel more depressed and fatigued. Poor posture also leads to tense muscles, which will also drain your energy. Most of the time we are unaware of the tension we hold in our back. If you put your arm out and make a tight fist, and hold it for 10 seconds, you will start to understand how much energy tight muscles use up. What you want to aim for is a posture that involves no tension, so that you are relaxed at all times of the day.

Poor posture restricts the blood flow so that eventually there is less oxygen reaching your cells and the blood is unable to nourish them; also, it squashes your abdominal organs, all of which will make you feel exhausted. Think about how you are sitting now. Are you slumped so that the area around your navel is compressed? Is there any tension in your back? Check to see if the bottom end of your breast-bone is lifted away from your abdomen. Just making this tiny correction will help. Aiming for better posture will definitely give you lots more energy.

The yoga postures or asanas will help to keep your spinal column and the cerebrospinal fluid healthy. The asanas also supply nutrients and fluids to your spinal discs. If they do not receive them, the discs become hard and start to degenerate. The spinal twists and backward bends described in later chapters will greatly help your back. As the yoga poses improve the strength of your spine, your breathing and digestion as well as your posture will improve. This in turn will improve your mental faculties – you will feel more energised and alert and your concentration will be better. For more information on perfect posture, see the Mountain Pose in Chapter 7.

Summary

As you will discover in the next chapter, yoga sees us as a whole being - not just a collection of individual parts. So, although I've talked about various parts - such as your digestive system, adrenal function, endocrine system and respiratory system - yoga aims to work on your whole system in order to bring everything back into balance, so that you can experience good health. Remember too that you need to work on achieving harmony and balance in your life - you need to balance work with relaxation and to eat properly. My recipe for combating fatigue is as follows:

- Practise the yoga postures given later - every day if possible.
- Take enough rest and relaxation.
- Eat a very nutritious diet and drink plenty of water.
- Practise the yoga breathing techniques given in Chapter 4. Check your own breathing rate.
- Sit outside in the sunshine when you can - we take in prana or energy from the food we eat, the air we breathe and from sunshine.
- Meditate for 20 minutes a day - see Chapter 11.
- Try and develop a positive attitude; set yourself goals in life so that you know in which direction you are going.

I hope this has given you a better insight into what may be causing your fatigue - and some suggestions for how to tackle the problem. In the following chapters, we will look more closely at yoga and see what it has to offer in terms of increasing your energy levels.

2 an introduction to yoga

The last chapter should have given you some idea about what is causing you to feel tired. In this chapter, I will introduce you to yoga and explain how it can help you to have much more vitality. Put simply, yoga will help you to beat fatigue, however it is caused, because yoga is all about using prana. Prana is the first unit of life force, or the energy that sustains all life. Prana is said to be the total of all the energy in the universe.

Although our bodies are saturated with prana (it is absorbed from the air, the sun and the food we eat), our vitality depends on how we are able to use this energy. Yoga will help you to control, direct and store prana. As you will discover later, yoga postures and exercises will help you to balance your own energy centres, or chakras, so that your prana can flow properly. Your chakras take in this universal energy via the nadis, which are channels like electric circuits. When your own energy is not flowing as it should, you become ill because prana cannot flow through the body. I'll be discussing prana and chakras in more detail in the next chapter, but for now you should understand that in yoga the traditional way for waking up this energy is through breath control, meditation and physical postures.

The Unity of Mind, Body and Spirit

Yoga is also about the balance of your physical, mental, emotional and spiritual states, and about how to bring these states into harmony. In yoga, we look at the whole system without trying to break the body up into separate parts. Your state of mind, for example, will affect your immune and endocrine (hormone) systems, which in turn will affect your circulation and breathing – and so on. In other words, it is impossible to look at any one part of the body in isolation. If you really want to beat fatigue and gain perfect health, you need to look at not just your physical requirements – which so much of Western living seems to concentrate on – but at your mental and spiritual needs as well. In this way, yoga sees a unity between mind, body and spirit. But what do we understand by 'mind', 'body' and 'spirit'? We place little importance on their interconnection. Most of us take too little exercise, suffer from an overload of stress and tension, and live in a society where the emphasis is on the material, not the spiritual.

Mind

According to Patanjali, an Indian sage who wrote about yoga around 2,000 years ago: 'Yoga is the control of thought waves of the mind'. This may surprise you if you thought yoga was just a series of exercises. In fact, Patanjali was making a very powerful statement. After all, an unquiet mind is very exhausting – it would be wonderful if you could learn how to control it. In yoga, a restless mind is likened to a chattering monkey, or the ripples on an otherwise calm lake. If you are mentally tense, you may suffer from racing thoughts, have a tendency to be over-emotional, or you may experience anxiety and phobias, even depression. All of this will deplete your energy. Practising yoga will put you back in the driving seat and help you to be calm and in control.

A thought *is* energy, and so how you think is very important for your health. Because you are what you think, working on the mind has a profound effect on the body. In yoga this is achieved through relaxation, concentration and visualisation exercises, learning to breathe properly and, ultimately, by meditation.

An example of how your mind can control your energy levels is demonstrated by the following experiment, which I have witnessed several times. It is used by Howard Kent, who ran the Yoga for Health Foundation in the UK and who is well known for having popularised yoga in the West in the early 1970s. He asks two volunteers to hold their arms out vertically. He then pushes on their arms to see how much resistance there is. One volunteer is then asked to think of 'nothing in particular', while the other is told to think of the mantra 'I breathe in life and energy' for one minute. Howard then pushes on the arms again. The arm of the person who has been thinking of nothing gives way easily, but the person who has been repeating the mantra finds he has the muscle strength to resist the pressure on his arm. So thinking positively can directly affect your muscle strength.

In another experiment – conducted when it was snowing outside – the central heating was turned off in Howard's office and the temperature fell to about 2°C. Howard was then wrapped in wet towels. His aim was to dry the towels with the heat of his body – which he did in about two and three-quarter hours. Most people would have suffered from hypothermia! When I asked him how and why he had done this, he said: 'I wanted to prove that the mind can control the body. All I did was to imagine I was lying in the hot sun. This shows that a mental image can be stronger than a physical "fact". It also shows how you can use the power of the mind to create your own reality.'

Body

Yoga postures help tremendously on a physical level because they both conserve and give energy – unlike ordinary exercise, such as jogging or aerobics, which actually uses up energy. Yoga helps your body because it:

- tones the muscles
- delays ageing
- benefits the joints and skeleton
- strengthens the circulation, heart and lung capacity – oxygenates the blood better and improves breathing
- improves digestion
- strengthens the back and makes the spine more flexible – so helps posture
- balances the nervous system – so helps to relax the whole body
- balances the endocrine system – so helps with hormone levels
- nourishes all organs and glands
- balances the chakras (your energy centres)
- cleanses and removes toxins
- gives energy.

Spirit

Spiritual balance is fundamental to yoga practice. Spirit can perhaps best be defined as being anything that is not physical - such as the abstract part of your being that you can nourish through love. To put this more simply, if you have a love of nature and of music or art, then you probably have an idea of what is spiritual. Living in the moment, or doing creative things like painting or listening to music, can help you to find this, because when you get lost in such tasks you are experiencing a universal unity. By this I mean that you forget your ego and connect with your real inner self. We will examine this in more detail when we look at meditation in Chapter 11.

A lack of spiritual direction can lead to depression, fear, anxiety and a loss of purpose in life. Listening in with yoga helps you to connect with your soul, spirit or inner self. It is about coming into balance with the Universal Life Force, or whatever you feel comfortable calling it. This will give you tremendous energy, for being spiritually depleted is very draining.

Listen in to the Rhythm of Your Body

Rhythm is fundamental to our wellbeing. Your body has its own rhythm: you have your own breathing rhythm, your own daily and monthly cycle (men as well as women), and your own heartbeat rhythm. If you think about it, the earth also has its own rhythm. There is the cycle of the seasons, the cycle of the moon and the cycle of day following night. This last cycle affects us profoundly. Our master gland, the hypothalamus - which is in the brain and controls many of our functions - actually secretes hormones depending on whether it is light or dark. Chronobiology, the science of looking at biological or carcadian rhythms, accepts that our bodies have an in-built rhythm of their own. As Dr Andrew Wright, medical advisor for the charity Action for ME, says: 'Health is dependent on the rhythmical changes of these in-built cycles imposing order on the body, thereby enforcing stability through change! Rhythms are so much a part of our lives, be they in music or dance or whatever, that it is not surprising that they play a part in keeping us well.'

Yoga is about self-awareness, and our awareness of natural rhythms is so often lost or numbed by the stresses in our current way of living. Our ancestors lived in harmony with the planet - they got up when the sun rose, went to bed at sunset, and ate local foods that were in season. Modern-day living has made us lose touch with these rhythms, so before you begin your yoga postures, it is important to develop this awareness.

Developing Awareness Exercise

This simple exercise involves no physical exertion.

- Ask yourself how you feel right now as you are reading this. Are you tired, interested, bored or energised? Do you feel well today? Now listen to the way you breathe and try to slow it down. Are you breathing only from the upper chest area? Is your heart beating fast or slow? Stop and think about this for a while.
- Start to think about the way you move. When you are walking up stairs, for example, try breathing in as you slowly lift your leg up, and out as you put it down. In this way you are starting to introduce rhythm into your movements - an awareness of how you move. You can also practise moving in time with your breath whenever you are out walking. Try breathing in as you walk for four steps, then out as you walk for four more steps.
- Consider what you eat. Do you buy local produce that is in season and - if possible - organic? Start to become more aware of yourself - how you actually feel (well, unwell, tired, happy, sad) - and start thinking about how you treat your body. Do you take your health for granted, eat lots of junk food and take little exercise, for example? As you start to notice yourself more by paying attention to your body and your health, you will start to develop inner awareness.

The Eight Limbs of Yoga

Yoga is very much about taking control and responsibility for your own health. As Patanjali explained, yoga is about controlling the mind. Patanjali saw illness as a state of imbalance that creates a negative energy, which in turn dims our prana, our life force. He said that this imbalance is created by things such as disease, sluggishness, carelessness, living in the world of illusion (i.e. not accepting things as they really are), sorrow, despair, anger; being miserable, and poor breathing. Of course, this is a never-ending cycle - if you are miserable and angry you won't have the energy to think positively! So Patanjali devised the Eight Limbs of Yoga to help break this cycle and achieve perfect health, ready for enlightenment. The eight limbs are as follows (with their Sanskrit names or English equivalent):

1 A code of universal ethics to be followed, known as the yamas
2 A code of personal conduct, called niyamas
3 The practice of physical postures, known as asanas
4 The practice and control of prana through yoga breathing - pranayama
5 The practice of learning to control and withdraw the senses
6 Concentration - learning to still the mind
7 Meditation
8 Enlightenment

Some people think of the Eight Limbs of Yoga as a ladder - or something that you learn in order of progression. This is not really true; all the limbs are important and form part of the whole concept of yoga. However, most people start yoga at step three and learn the postures that exercise the body and relax the mind. After regular practice of this, and perhaps step four - breath control - you will realise other changes are happening. Your attitude to life will start to shift as you become more balanced and in harmony with your true self. This may then lead you on to examine steps one and two - the yamas and niyamas. You may find that you start to become more thoughtful and compassionate and less ruled by your desires, and so you move on to step five - the withdrawal of your senses. As your concentration becomes better and your mind calmer, you are ready for meditation.

In this book, because we are dealing specifically with fatigue, we will be concentrating on the third limb (the yoga postures), the fourth limb (yoga breathing) and the seventh limb (meditation).

Asanas - the Yoga Postures

The third limb of yoga comprises the yoga postures, or asanas. This is how most people think of yoga - as a form of exercise - but really the asanas are much more than that. I've already listed benefits these postures can give, such as balancing muscles, joints, glands, nerves and organs, as well as reducing fatigue and helping to soothe and discipline the mind and keep the body free from disease. But the postures are not exercise in the way we generally understand exercise - they are not something that should cause you great exertion or strain. Unlike most forms of exercise, yoga is non-competitive - you work at your own pace without worrying about how more advanced anyone else may be.

One of the first things yoga postures do is to stretch everything, and stretching is amazingly beneficial: it relieves tiredness and tension, loosens tight muscles and encourages the release of endorphins - the body's natural tranquillisers.

Yoga postures are always practised in conjunction with your breathing - for example, you breathe in as you lift a limb, and out as you lower it. In this way, you learn to do things more slowly, in rhythm with your breath. You will gain better breath control and achieve greater body awareness as you learn to co-ordinate your movements.

When you learn the yoga postures, you will also learn how to relax properly in the Pose of Complete Rest. It is said that this posture is the most difficult to learn because most of us find it very difficult to let everything go! Don't ever feel guilty about practising relaxation. Yoga is about who you are - and not about what you do. So, do give yourself time to relax after a yoga session - and between the postures if you need to. Relaxation will help recharge your batteries and release new energy. It will overcome any exhaustion brought about by stress. It also clears blockages at a deep level so healing can take place.

I have witnessed how relaxation can undo tension on many occasions, when people have broken down and cried during a yoga relaxation class. This is because they had been holding on to tension and grief for many years, and the relaxation then started to unblock their energy centres and release stress so that they could experience their true emotions again. I'm not suggesting that when you practise the relaxation exercise you will break down, but the release of feelings can start to put you back in control of yourself again. Yoga will help you to bring about peace of mind. As years of tension start to shift, you will find yourself able to listen in more and take control – and you will discover much more energy! This will take practice – most of us go through our lives not even aware that we are tense much of the time. It's only by practising relaxation every day that you will start to realise the difference between being tense and being relaxed. Once you have gained this awareness, however, you can use it outside your yoga session, so that if anything does make you stressed, you can consciously relax.

The Pose of Complete Rest (Savasana)

- Lie down on the floor or on your bed with your eyes closed. Keep your legs slightly apart and your palms facing upwards. Wriggle your heels down so that your feet fall away from your hips and relax apart. Stretch your hands down to lengthen the space between your neck and shoulders.
- Now take yourself through each part of your body, tensing each muscle group then relaxing. Starting with your feet, tense all the muscles in your toes, feet and ankles, then relax them. Now squeeze the muscles in your legs – your calf and thigh muscles – as tightly as possible and lift your legs up slightly from your support. Hold for a few seconds, then relax. Pull your tummy muscles in, then relax. Hold your arms out and make fists with your hands, then relax them. Lift your shoulders up towards your ears, then relax them downwards. Think about any tension in your back and shoulders and allow it to ease away as you sink into your support. Now squeeze your face together as tightly as possible, then relax. Feel your jaw relax and the space between your eyebrows ease, and imagine someone is massaging your scalp so that all the tension in your face and head disappears.
- Try to relax as much as possible. Feel your whole body grow heavy as it sinks into your support – there is no need for you to hold on to any tension at all. Pay particular attention to your jaw, shoulders, back and stomach – the areas where you carry most stress. Slow your breathing rate down and visualise releasing tension on each out-breath.

I would suggest that you try to practise the Pose of Complete Rest every day. When you stretch a muscle, this helps it to relax more when you let it go, although eventually you will be able to do the relaxation sequence without having to tense your muscles first. If you don't have much time, do this pose before you go to sleep. As you practise more, you will start to learn how your body feels when it is relaxed compared to how it feels when tense. You can then carry this awareness with you into everyday situations so that if you are under stress, you can consciously drop your shoulders, unlock your jaw and slow down your breathing. This is a very powerful tool to help you cope with tension, one of the causes of fatigue.

Pranayama - The Control of Energy through Yoga Breathing

Pranayama is the fourth limb of yoga. Prana, as already discussed, means universal energy or life force, and pranayama is the process of directing, controlling and storing this energy in the body using yoga breathing techniques. The word pranayama actually means control of prana or life-force energy.

How you breathe profoundly affects your health and emotions. If you are angry or tense, for example, you will probably breathe rapidly from the upper part of your chest area, which means you won't be using your diaphragm. This also works the other way round. In other words, if under normal circumstances you breathe quite fast and only from your chest, this will eventually affect your thoughts and emotions. You may become agitated, depressed and anxious because your body is not receiving the correct combination of oxygen and carbon dioxide. Your concentration may slow down. And this will make you very fatigued. It is said in yoga that one outburst of anger uses up three months' supply of energy! If you are constantly under pressure, shallow breathing may become your normal way of life, even when the stress has passed. Because your state of mind is controlled by the way you breathe, it stands to reason that you can reverse this process and control your mind by taking charge of your breathing. Most of us don't take much notice of how we breathe - it is an unconscious action. Pranayama exercises will show you how to become more aware of this.

Taking control of your breathing can lead to a state of deep calmness. It is said in yoga that we are allotted only a certain number of breaths in life - so a person with rapid, shallow breathing may live a shorter life than someone who breathes slowly and deeply. Proper breathing cleanses the system, refreshes and invigorates the mind, increases alertness and concentration, and can renew the subtle energy body (your aura) so that healing can happen. It helps promote deeper sleep, relieves tension, improves digestion, lowers blood pressure, slows the heartbeat and generally leads to a more contented state of being. Those are a lot of reasons to make pranayama part of your everyday routine!

Breathing Exercise

- Lie on the floor or on the bed, on your back. First of all, tune in to your breathing rhythm. Is your breathing fast or slow? Try to slow it down so that you breathe in for a count of four, then out to a count of four. This is one cycle. Using a clock or watch with a second hand, time yourself and try to do around 10-12 cycles a minute. (Although this is the rate to aim for, it is not important at this stage if your breathing rate is higher.)
- Now put your hands on your solar plexus (just above your navel). Breathe in: you should feel the movement of your diaphragm as your lungs inflate and swell into your abdominal cavity. Try to keep your abdomen firm at this point.
- Now move your hands one hand width up so they are on the lower part of your ribcage. Your whole ribcage should move up and down as you breathe, with your hands moving up and out as you breathe in, and down as you breathe out. Let your diaphragm rise unrestricted as you breathe. To emphasise this action, put your hands around your ribcage with your thumbs to the back and your fingers to the front. As you breathe in, feel your ribcage expand upwards and outwards. Squeeze it in gently as you breathe out.

Start to get used to the difference between your in-breath and your out-breath, and try to develop an awareness of your diaphragm when you breathe, so that you never breathe just from your upper chest. Practise this twice a day for five minutes - perhaps when you wake up and just before you go to sleep. As you get used to this way of breathing, incorporate it in your daily routine - whether you are sitting or standing. Check yourself several times a day. Are you still breathing using your diaphragm? Does your breathing need to be slower? If you are ever in a stressful situation, such as an argument, consciously slow down your breathing. You will be amazed at how much calmer and in control you feel.

Meditation

There are many reasons why meditation, the seventh limb of yoga, is important. Meditation calms and heals the mind and gives a huge boost of energy that is as refreshing - if not more so - than sleep. And meditation can also help you to develop your spiritual awareness and find your own truth: who you really are and what your purpose in life is. If you are not interested in your spiritual development and you are reading this book only to discover more energy, you will still find meditation an invaluable tool for fighting fatigue. Meditation is a state of mind where your brain rhythms actually slow down. This happens when you sit still, with your spine upright and your brain clear of all thoughts. It's rather like looking at a blank cinema screen - you still your mind. Howard Kent used the analogy of a car engine: most of us are using the engine with a foot on the throttle, but when we meditate we take the foot off, and the engine - or mind - just ticks over.

Personally, I have experienced very deep peace and stillness through meditation, and it has enabled me to get through many crises, including the death of a close member of my family. It takes time and perseverance to learn, and you must be disciplined enough to make 20 minutes free for meditation every day - but the benefits are well worth the effort. There is more about how to meditate in Chapter 11.

The Yoga Diet

In the last chapter you may have begun to realise that diet plays a vital role in energy production. If you are tired, stressed or suffering from a condition such as depression or hypoglycaemia what you eat will affect you greatly. Most people don't realise that diet forms part of yoga. I've talked about prana or life-force energy, and in yoga, eating the right food is one of the major ways to obtain this.

You may remember that in yoga you get your energy from the sun, air, soil and water. One of the most effective ways your body can get energy is from the metabolism of food. The storehouse for prana in your body is believed to be in your solar plexus (your navel area, where digestion takes place), so good food is vital for good health. Think of your food as medicine – if you want energy then you must eat food of quality. If you eat food of poor quality, you will feel fatigued and unwell. When you are tired, it is more tempting to eat quick, ready-prepared meals – but this is the time when you really need to pay more attention to your diet than ever before.

The first thing to understand is that food also has a vital energy force. In order to benefit from this food-energy, you have to eat food in as near to its natural state as possible. This is because food that has just been picked has much more prana. So whenever possible, eat only whole foods that have not undergone processing in any way. Ideally, you should pick a home-grown vegetable and eat it on the spot! This isn't always possible, but food that has been stored too long on the supermarket shelf or in your fridge; food that has been sprayed with pesticides or treated with hormones and antibiotics; food that is overcooked or left over from the day before will not have any prana that your body can use. These processes destroy the potential of the food you eat and actually deplete rather than increase your energy. Your diet should therefore include organic whole grains and pulses, fresh fruit and vegetables, eggs, beans, live yoghurt, nuts and seeds.

In yoga, it is believed that a pure diet purifies the mind, so the food you choose should be simple, sweet-smelling, light, nutritious and easily digestible. If you do eat meat, try to find organic or free-range products. The stress an animal experiences in an abattoir is very prana-depleting, and its fear is passed on through stress hormones in its meat. If you are going to follow the path of yoga strictly, you might choose not to eat meat at all, as this is contrary to the guidance given in the first limb of yoga (yama), which advises non-harm to any living being (ahimsa). Another reason for not eating meat is that if you eat the flesh of any living being, you are gaining your prana second-hand (the animal got the energy first-hand from the soil).

So think about what you eat. Rather than cooking pre-packaged meat and vegetables that have been stored on a supermarket shelf, try to eat organic foods in season.

There is a reason for this. In the winter; root vegetables can help you get more energy from the earth at a time when you are getting less from the sun. Try to eat local produce that won't have been spoilt by travelling and storage. Eat three nutritious meals a day - including breakfast - and if you have snacks, make sure that they are of good quality, such as seeds and nuts. Try to cut out all sugar and sweet foods, as these will ultimately make you feel more fatigued. Drink alcohol in moderation - and if you have candida or hypoglycaemia, avoid it altogether. Do not embark on a calorie-controlled diet as this will seriously curtail your nutritional and energy intake. If you are eating proper nutritious food, you don't need to diet. As you practise yoga, you will eventually attain your ideal weight.

Preferred Foods

In yoga, the foods you should eat are known as Sattivic, which means food that is easy to digest, gives lots of energy, and helps to purify the system and calm the mind. Try to include as much of the following in your diet as you can:

- organic fruit and vegetables grown locally and in season
- whole grains such as brown rice and sprouted wheat
- pulses such as chickpeas, soya beans and lentils
- seeds such as sunflower; pumpkin and sesame
- fresh nuts (not peanuts)
- milk (used traditionally in yoga as a source of protein)
- plain live yoghurt
- honey as a sweetener
- bottled or filtered water
- herbal teas.

If all this sounds too difficult, remember that yoga is about following the middle path - in other words, not doing anything too extreme. However; you do need to work towards a basically healthy diet before you can allow yourself the odd treat!

Finally, in yoga it is believed that much of the prana in food is absorbed through the tongue. So chew your food very thoroughly before you swallow - it should be like a fine paste. This will also help with your digestion: the nutrients are more easily absorbed into the bloodstream so you are less likely to develop food intolerances and won't use up so much energy digesting your food. Relax and sit down when you eat - we saw in the last chapter how stress leads to poor digestion because the digestive process slows right down when you are under pressure. Try not to drink water when you eat, as this will dilute the digestive juices. Eat only when you are hungry, and then only in moderation.

Ideally, if you are eating good food which has been grown in soil of reasonable quality, you shouldn't need to take supplements. If you are suffering from fatigue, however, it is possible that your digestive tract is not absorbing all the nutrients, especially if you suffer from candida. You could try taking vitamin C, a B-vitamin complex, calcium and magnesium and evening primrose oil. Because we all have individual requirements, you may like to consider visiting a nutritional therapist for more advice.

Water

You've probably heard this before - you need to drink lots of water! Your body needs lots of lubrication so that everything can function - from circulation and elimination through to the working of all your organs. A yoga teacher cited the analogy of a car battery to me - unless your car battery is topped up with purified water, the engine won't function. So it is with your body - if you don't drink between one-and-a-half to two litres of water a day, your body will not function as it should and you will feel fatigued.

What Yoga Really Means

I hope this chapter has given you an idea of how yoga can help you. The word 'yoga' means to unite, and this is what yoga is about - helping us to unite with the infinite, or universe. In yoga, we are seen as having a real self - which is hidden away under our ego and wants and desires. If you can rediscover your real self, this will help you to experience your connection to everything in the universe, which will give you tremendous energy. Yoga isn't a religion, but it is a philosophy - a way of life that can help you discover your own path to health and vitality.

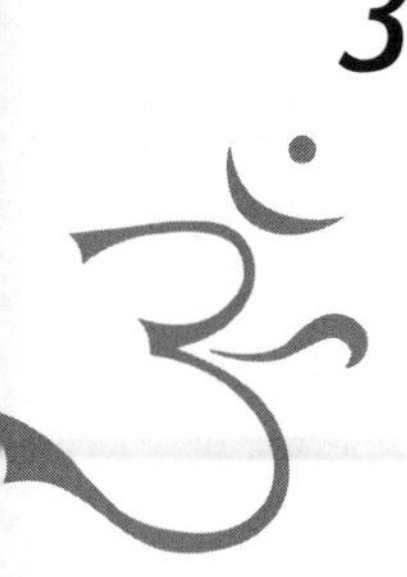

3 energy and your energy centres

In this chapter, I'm going to talk about energy or prana in more detail, and show how working with it is fundamental to your vitality and health. If you understand prana, then you will be able to make better use of it, particularly if you use the yoga breathing techniques (pranayama) in the next chapter.

Prana – The Universal Energy Force

In the Introduction, I said that prana is a kind of cosmic energy and is thought to be the sum of all the energy in the universe. The ancient yogis believed that this energy has no chemical or physical form, but is our true nourishment. We take prana into our bodies via our nadis, subtle energy channels which feed our chakras, or energy centres. I shall explain nadis and chakras in more detail later on, but for now I want to try and give you a better idea of what prana is. Interestingly, modern science is now coming to the same conclusion as the ancient yogis of India who discovered and worked with prana – that there is some form of Universal Energy Force!

Let's compare a couple of views on this. The writer Andre van Lysebeth proposes that prana may be electromagnetic, or at least composed partly of electrically charged particles. Following this theory through, he suggests that certain locations – such as mountainous regions and the seaside – have more prana because they are highly charged with negative ions. To me this makes sense – I certainly feel invigorated when I am skiing or near the sea. Howard Kent from the Yoga for Health Foundation said: 'The constituent parts of prana are not yet wholly understood, but clearly include oxygen, the electromagnetic force and probably negative and positive ions.' These two yoga experts agree that prana includes all forces of nature known to man, including gravity, light, heat, electricity, magnetism, the nervous system and the mind.

In quantum physics, everything that exists in the universe is seen as having patterns of energy - of which atoms are a part. For example, if two atoms merge they have incredible energy - enough to power a small town. I am not talking about fusing or splitting atoms here; I use this only as an example to show how much energy exists in even the smallest particle in the universe and to explain that these particles are in constant motion - that is, they are moving in patterns of energy.

The Theory of Relativity shows that mass has nothing to do with a substance, but is a form of energy. So every tiny particle in the universe is not a static object but a process involving energy, which manifests as the particle's mass. That includes you! Put simply, this means that you - and every object you can think of - are a mass of vibrating bits of energetic particles. This is quite amazing if you think about it! It's even more incredible if you understand that you can learn how to use this tremendous energy through yoga.

Three hundred years ago, the physicist Sir Isaac Newton saw all these particles as separate, and it is only recently that science has discovered that all matter is interconnected, interrelated and interdependent. At the beginning of the 20th century, for example, the physicist Niels Bohr showed that all particles in the universe are constantly 'in touch' with each other - informing one another of what is happening. So particles are actually entangled, forming a huge cosmic web of interacting particles. This brings us on to the unity I talked about in Chapter 2, when I said that the aim of yoga is to help us realise that we are not separate, but united and part of everything. Because all particles in the universe are connected and related, each one influences everything else. It is said that if a butterfly flaps its wings, the effect will be felt on the most distant star. So imagine how your actions affect everything in the universe!

What I am saying is that our universe does have a unity - of which we are part - and it also has energy, even if it seems to be an inanimate mass. This energy is prana - and prana is our link to the universe. By using yoga techniques, prana can be controlled, directed and stored at will. If you can learn to tap in to prana, you can have access to limitless energy! You will learn some of these techniques when we look at the special breathing techniques in Chapter 4, but meanwhile here are some suggestions to help you maximise your supply of prana, the universal energy force.

- Try to walk barefoot on the ground at least once a day to benefit from the earth's natural electric field. Recent scientific research has found that we may have a sixth sense which responds to the earth's magnetic field; an organ which detects changes in geomagnetic fields has been found in fish, and it is thought humans may have this too. Renewing contact with the earth is particularly important if you have been travelling - cars, trains and aeroplanes act as a Faraday cage (an environment which prevents electromagnetic energy from passing through) and consequently block out the earth's natural prana. This is one reason why travelling can be so tiring.
- If possible, don't spend too much time in buildings or structures made of metal. Again, this is because of the Faraday cage effect and the need to 'ground' with the earth's magnetic field, which is beneficial to health.
- Try to avoid air conditioning, smoke, dust and pollution. These are enemies of prana. If you live in a town, try to spend as much time in the country as you can. I know this isn't always possible, but at least be aware of your environment.
- Sunbathe sensibly, when possible, to increase your intake of solar prana. As with all things in yoga, do this in moderation.
- Get as much fresh air as possible. Use an ionizer in your home if you can, especially if you live with a smoker.
- Avoid using plastic or synthetic materials; they attract positive ions and reduce prana. Try to store food in paper or glass, and to wear only natural fibres such as cotton or silk.
- Most important of all, remember that prana is raised by positive thinking - especially if you direct it with awareness - because the mind is in part prana. The guided visualisations in the next section on chakras will help you do this.
- Finally, yoga postures, good food, sunlight, fresh air, correct breathing techniques and meditation can all encourage prana to flow.

Now we shall look at nadis, the channels that enable you to take in prana from the universe to feed your chakras and your whole system.

Nadis - Your Energy Channels

The word 'nadi' means a channel or tube. Nadis are the conductors of prana; in other words, they are channels for the circulation of vital energy. There are said to be at least 72,000 nadis that are related to our body. Some yoga experts have said that nadis are like our nerves, but others disagree. The best way to explain is to say that nadis are very similar to the subtle energy channels known as meridians in Chinese medicine. I like to think of nadis as electric currents that enable prana to be taken in from the universe, giving energy to the material body. In a radio set analogy, prana would be the radio waves and our chakras the aerials that pick them up and circulate them round the body via the nadis, the electrical circuits.

Practising yoga helps to keep the nadis open, so that maximum energy or prana can flow. Certain yoga breathing techniques do this effectively and are very energising. For example, Alternate Nostril Breathing works on the major nadis, and this in turn helps to purify the whole network of nadis.

The three major nadis I want to talk about relate to the spine and nostrils. I have explained that we have our own electromagnetic field, and it is important that you know that yoga has always recognised this kind of energy, long before electricity was discovered. For example, in yoga, polarity - or negative and positive - is a very important concept because it involves the balance of the complete whole. The physical postures in yoga are sometimes referred to as Hatha yoga. 'Hatha' means sun (ha) and moon (tha) - in other words, it incorporates the two opposite ideas of day and night. In yoga, it is believed that the left nostril carries the nadi which is the moon, or feminine energy, and relates to the negative pole. The right nostril carries the nadi which is the sun, or masculine, positive energy. They intertwine and descend along the spine, the main nadi. The spine is so important in yoga because it carries vital energy to feed the main chakras. So good posture really will help your energy levels.

The Chakras - Your Energy Centres

As we have already seen, yoga understands prana as the basic source of life energy, and the body takes in energy via nadis to a series of centres called chakras. Understanding your chakras will help you to understand and explore your own energy. There are many chakras in the body, but I will concentrate on the main seven, which run parallel with your spine. These chakras vibrate with a particular frequency, which also relates to sound and colour. If your energy becomes blocked and a chakra is not vibrating as it should be, you become out of balance, and ill health and fatigue will follow.

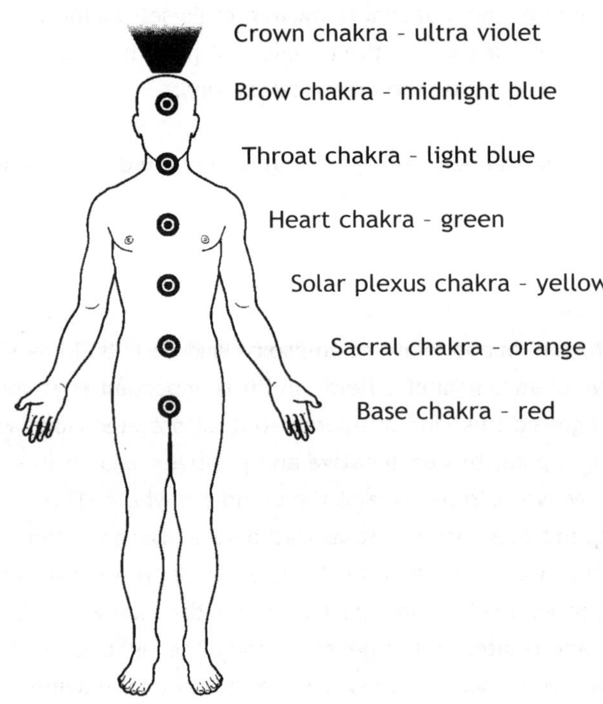

The Chakras

In Sanskrit, chakra means a wheel or vortex - and that is what a chakra is, a spinning vortex which takes in energy to feed all areas of the human system: your physical and your subtle body ('subtle' is the yogic term for our energy field). Chakras work on a physical, emotional and spiritual level and each one relates to a particular area of the body. Although I will be talking about each chakra separately later on, it's important to understand that they are all related. We can't really understand our individual chakras without looking at all of them. At the end of this chapter, I will give you two exercises to help balance all your chakras. The chakras have Sanskrit names but to make things simple I shall refer to them by their English names. The seven main chakras are as follows, with the first five all located along the spine:

- The Root or Base Chakra, at the bottom of the spine, with the funnel pointing downwards to bring up energy from the earth.
- The Sacral Chakra, between the pubic bone and the navel.
- The Solar Plexus Chakra, located at the navel.
- The Heart Chakra, just to the right of the heart.
- The Throat Chakra, at the throat.
- The Brow Chakra, just above the point between the eyebrows.
- The Crown Chakra, just above the top of the head, with the funnel pointing upwards to take in energy from above.

Your chakras are like energy stepping stones - as you work up to your higher energy centres towards the Crown Chakra, the vibration rate increases. You may remember that when I was explaining prana I said every particle and atom in the universe vibrates with energy. This vibration happens at different frequencies. For example, light has a much higher electromagnetic vibration than sound. So each chakra vibrates and each chakra transmits energy from one level to another; distributing pranic energy to your physical body. The lower chakras relate to your more earth-bound, emotional states and the higher ones to your spiritual state.

Your chakras can exist in two states: open or blocked. They can also become closed, but that only happens when you die. To put it simply, just remember that if your chakra is blocked it is taking in less prana, and if it is too open it may be taking in more energy than you are able to cope with. For example, after a bereavement, grief may open your

Heart Chakra too quickly to passionate emotions, which may be overwhelming. On the other hand, if you try to ignore the feelings of grief and deny your emotions, you will eventually block the energy of the Heart Chakra. Blocked chakras can lead to distorted thinking and perception, anger and neurosis, or the over-use of defence mechanisms such as repression and being out of touch with your feelings. This eventually leads to physical ailments that relate to the specific chakras. It is important, therefore, that as you listen in more to yourself using yoga, you learn the lessons your chakras show you and don't try to block any emotional pain or experience. Otherwise you will become ill. Losing your energy may be the first clue that this is happening.

I'm now going to talk about each chakra in more detail so that you will have a better idea of which particular area you need to work on. As I've indicated, each chakra relates to a colour, emotion and physical area of your body. The first four also have related elements. I'll also explain what can happen if the chakra is too open or closed. At the end of each section there are exercises for you to try. Details of specific yoga postures which will help you to work on each chakra are given in Chapters 5-8.

The Root Chakra

- At the physical level, your Root Chakra relates to your adrenal system, your lower bowel and your system of elimination.
- The Root Chakra vibrates as the colour red. It is represented by the element of earth and consequently has a solid, dense frequency.
- Emotionally, the Root is your anchor and foundation chakra. It is about being in the real material world, being grounded in the here and now. It is also associated with the will to live and wanting to be alive – the sense of 'I am here!'
- A blocked Root Chakra can leave you lacking in energy, with a weak constitution and a feeling of being depersonalised. You may feel you are not really here; you may live in your head too much; or you may indulge in excessive daydreaming. It can also lead to a fear of letting go and opening up to your inner creativity. Having a blocked Root Chakra can be likened to a tent with insecurely attached guy ropes, making the structure unsound.
- If your Root Chakra is too open, you may be so grounded in the 'here and now' that you lose touch with your spiritual horizons and become very materialistic.

- If the Root Chakra is balanced, you will be able to accept yourself, your body and your life as they are and consequently enjoy a feeling of security, confidence and self-esteem. Your energy and enthusiasm for life emanate from this chakra when it is vibrating correctly.

Susie's Story

I worked in a large university library and was also researching for my PhD. I always used to put a lot of pressure on myself to work hard - and I suppose I am quite cerebral; I would rather read a book than play a game of tennis! About three years ago, I had a nervous breakdown. It started with panic attacks - I would wake up in the middle of the night unable to breathe or swallow, with my heart pounding so fast that I thought I was going to have a heart attack. I would also feel very faint and, most frightening of all, I felt unreal, as if I wasn't really there. I was tired all the time - so exhausted, in fact, that I could hardly work. I grew more and more afraid - of what I don't really know, but everything made me so fearful that I became suicidal. I lost all my confidence and thought I was a terrible person - a complete failure. I felt as if my whole life was slipping out of my control and I physically tensed my whole body to try to hold on. My doctor prescribed Valium and antidepressants, which just made me more tired. To cut a long story short, I got worse and couldn't leave my house without panicking. I was referred to a private psychiatric hospital. I thought it would be terrible there but it was brilliant. They had a yoga class every day, which I joined - and to my amazement I started to feel better, more 'here' if you know what I mean. The yoga teacher taught me some breathing techniques and explained how to control my breathing so that I didn't hyperventilate. She suggested I did some work on my Root Chakra and showed me how to ground myself using visualisation. I also took up pottery in hospital - and gardening, which I found very soothing. When I was well enough I was discharged from hospital, and I then decided to put my research work on hold while I retrained as a landscape gardener. I now spend lots of time working outside. I also do about half an hour of yoga every day and I belong to a group which I go to once a week. Yoga has helped to ground me; it made me realise that there are more important things in life than getting qualifications - but best of all it has given me boundless energy!

Exercises to Balance the Root Chakra

The Root Chakra faces downwards from the base of the spine to take in energy from the earth. These suggestions are to help you get back in touch with yourself using this energy, and for this reason they include visualisation but not meditation. Meditation is excellent for balancing the upper chakras, but if you think your Root Chakra is blocked, leave meditation until you feel more grounded. Remember, it is vital for the health of all your chakras to have the Root Chakra balanced. Like a tree, the deeper your roots, the further your branches can reach out to the sunlight.

VISUALISATION

Sit cross-legged so that your spine is in contact with the floor. Close your eyes and visualise a ray of red light coming up through the floor into your spine on an in-breath. On the out-breath, breathe the colour into your whole body so that you are bathed in a red energising light. Really think about the colour. Imagine what it might smell and taste like. Imagine that you have become the colour red. Now look around the room. Be aware of everything in the room. Look at the ceiling, the walls and the furniture. Notice any ornaments, objects or books. Feel the texture of this book that you are holding. Listen for any sounds. Can you smell anything in the room? Rub your hands together and be aware of yourself in the room. Now stand up, keeping your back as straight as possible, your shoulders relaxed and your head lifted. Imagine red roots going down from your feet into the floor and through into the ground, taking in nourishment and energy from the earth.

YOGA POSTURES

To select postures for the Root Chakra, you need to look at anything that gets the base of the spine in contact with the ground. Try the Sitting Forward Stretch, the Boat and the Sitting Twist, which you will find in Chapters 5-8. The Pose of Complete Rest is also excellent for this chakra.

OTHER WAYS

Anything that gets you in contact with the earth or helps you to be in the 'here and now' of the material world is beneficial. Walking, gardening, dancing or creative pursuits such as pottery are all excellent. Try walking barefoot across the grass - or just sitting in the garden appreciating the beauty of nature and the wonder of creation. You can also try wearing red clothes - such as socks, trousers or skirts - below the waist (i.e. near the Root Chakra).

The Sacral Chakra

- The Sacral Chakra is associated with your reproductive system, including the ovaries and uterus, the testes and the prostate. It is also responsible for the bladder and kidneys. Infertility, vaginal and pelvic infections, premenstrual syndrome (PMS), endometriosis, impotence or prostatic diseases may indicate that this chakra is out of balance. Many of these ailments can also cause fatigue.
- This chakra is represented by the element of water and the colour orange.
- At an emotional level, your Sacral Chakra is about the creation of life; it also relates to your sensual side and how you convey this to others. Therefore if this chakra is blocked, it may show as a disruption in sexual relations with your partner.
- A Sacral Chakra that is too open can lead to envy, lust, fear; confusion or over-dependence on your partner.
- The Sacral Chakra is also concerned with the balance between female and male - yin (female) and yang (male) in Chinese philosophy, or Ha Tha in Sanskrit. Therefore, when the Sacral Chakra is balanced, you can be independent and whole and contribute to the balance within an interdependent relationship.

Exercises to Balance the Sacral Chakra

VISUALISATION

Lie on the floor and relax everything as much as possible. Close your eyes and imagine that you are walking barefoot through a wood. Smell the fragrant, energising scent of the pine trees and of the woodland flowers that grow next to the path. Feel the texture of the wood mulch under your feet. In the distance you can hear a stream babbling. Walk towards the sound. You see a fast-running brook filled with amber water. Imagine you are cupping your hands together and filling them with the golden liquid. Hold the water to your mouth and drink it. Feel the colour amber lighting up your whole body and giving you energy as you drink the liquid.

Now walk downstream. You come across a large pond, where the water has been dammed. The water looks mysterious and deep - but inviting.

You take off all your clothes and immerse yourself in the warm water. Imagine you are lying on your back for a while and just floating as the water soothes, purifies and caresses you. When you get out of the water, tell yourself you are now refreshed and revitalised.

YOGA POSTURES
Yoga postures for the Sacral Chakra include pelvic exercises such as the Pelvic Tilt. Other excellent postures are the Cat and the Locust.

The Solar Plexus Chakra

- At the physical level, your Solar Plexus Chakra relates to your pancreas, stomach, liver, gall bladder; spleen and your small intestine. Eating disorders, hypoglycaemia, diabetes, pancreatic problems, indigestion and irritable bowel syndrome may be associated with this chakra being unbalanced.
- The Solar Plexus Chakra is represented by the element of fire and the colour yellow.
- Your Solar Plexus Chakra is your true energy centre, also known as your inner fire or sun centre. One of the reasons for this is that you get your stamina by the process of digesting food. The right food is considered very important in yoga because it provides the energy for maintaining life, and can certainly help you to beat fatigue!
- Your Solar Plexus Chakra is also the centre for your major emotions, your ambitions, your wants and desires. It is your ego centre. If the Root Chakra is where you are grounded in the physical world and the sense of 'to be', your Solar Plexus Chakra is your centre of 'I am'. From this comes the expression that someone is very 'centred', referring to how they are in relation to other people. One of the most energy-depleting experiences is to live your life through others and experience other people's emotions, rather than having clear boundaries between yourself and those around you.

- If this chakra is too open, it can act as an antenna that may pick up the negative energy of others too quickly. You may also be over-emotional, greedy, angry or aggressive. Or you may become a 'people pleaser', always thinking of other people's feelings but never looking after your own needs properly. This can make you overly submissive, passive and powerless, which can lead to resentment and real exhaustion.
- If your Solar Plexus Chakra is too closed, you may have the opposite experience and become selfish and unfeeling. Lack of drive and willpower, an inability to project yourself in the world, depression, exhaustion and stress are all associated with a blocked Solar Plexus.
- For a healthy Solar Plexus Chakra, you need to learn to separate your own emotions and responsibilities from other people's, to be open to experiences and not block your feelings. When we looked at the section on stress, we saw how stored emotions cause tension and exhaustion. Because this chakra relates to your emotions, often you can actually feel tension around this area if you have an emotional upset. For example, if you have a shock, you may have the physical feeling that you have been punched in the stomach. If something makes you frightened or anxious, you are probably going to have 'butterflies in your tummy'. When your Solar Plexus Chakra is balanced, you will feel centred and confident, and you will be flexible rather than rigid in your thinking. You will be able to show your emotions, but you will be in control of these emotions, rather than the other way around. This will give you tremendous confidence and energy.

Exercises to Balance the Solar Plexus Chakra

VISUALISATIONS

- If you feel that other people drain you, try imagining a mirror placed between you and them. Any negative energy they give out is therefore reflected back to them, rather than absorbed by you. Any positive energy that you give out is reflected back to you so that they are unable to drain off your vitality.
- Another excellent visualisation is to imagine a white light surrounding you. This will protect you from negative energies.

- Lie on the floor and relax as much as possible. Now breathe in and out slowly from your ribcage area, using your diaphragm. Try and slow down your breathing. Imagine you can feel the sun warming your abdomen. You are breathing the golden globe of the sun into your sun centre - your Solar Plexus Chakra. Feel this warm golden light emanating from this centre, filling the rest of your body with yellow-gold energy and vitality.

YOGA POSTURES

The Bow and the Boat are good postures for balancing the Solar Plexus Chakra. One of the most beneficial postures in yoga for dealing with negative emotions, particularly anger, is the Woodchopper.

The Heart Chakra

- At the physical level, your Heart Chakra relates to your blood and circulation, your heart, lungs and your thymus gland. A blocked Heart Chakra can lead to heart problems and, because of its association with the thymus gland, problems with your immune function.
- The Heart Chakra is represented by the colour green and the element of air.
- Your emotions rise from your Solar Plexus Chakra to your Heart Chakra, where they are translated into the higher feelings of love, harmony and compassion. This includes love and openness for yourself as well as for others. Unconditional love flows through this chakra - for mankind and all living beings - and helps you to see only the good in others.
- If your Heart Chakra is too open, you may be too sensitive and over-concerned with others' needs. All your love and compassion will flow out towards others, which will make you very exhausted.
- If this chakra is blocked, you may have a problem in maintaining loving relationships. For example, you might see others as hostile and threatening, rather than kind and giving. If you ever feel that you are cold, ruthless and detached from others or from your own feelings, you probably need to do some work with this chakra.

- As with all your chakras, your Heart Chakra needs to be balanced so that your energy can flow; if you are over emotional or have difficulty showing your emotions, you will feel fatigued and physically drained because this energy is blocked.

Emma's Story

I've always had difficulty in expressing my emotions. As a child I was told not to cry and that it was wrong to complain about anything. I suppose in the end I became very detached from everything – I even remember not being able to cry when my mother died.

I used to feel as if I was acting a role in life, somehow not really connected to anything. I was very ambitious and worked my way up to Head of Human Resources in a large retail company.

I married and had two children. Of course I loved them, but I found it very difficult to show them any real affection – I was never one to cuddle or touch a lot. I found trying to hold down my job and run a family unbelievably tiring. My husband works abroad a lot, so in a way I was like a single parent, trying to work hard and deal with the children on my own. The house was always in a mess and inevitably backup support such as part-time nannies and cleaners let me down.

I suppose I resented my life, but at the time I never actually stopped to question how I felt – I was too busy trying to run everything smoothly for everyone else and work hard to pay our huge mortgage. I was Super Woman, in charge of everything – from organising school runs, managing the house and doing the shopping and cooking, to holding down a full-time job. I used to joke that the only time I had to myself was in the car on the way to work or in the bathroom!

In the end I felt like a wrung-out dishcloth with absolutely no spark of energy – I was just getting through every day as best I could. I joined an aerobics class to see if I could get more energy, but that just became something else on my list I that had to fit in. I started having problems at work; my manager was always criticising me and made an official complaint that I was cold and unfeeling towards those I dealt with. I was so run down that I got ill with really bad angina attacks, but this turned out to be a blessing in disguise because it slowed me down and made me start to assess what I wanted in life.

I took a month off work, and my husband and I decided to move to a smaller house so that I could work part-time. I then joined a yoga class, which was a real turning point. I started to meditate every day and really enjoyed the sense of calm it gave me. Meditation helped me to connect with my real self at last. I thought of meditation as my time, my 'treat'; it was never another thing on a list to do. My yoga teacher suggested I keep a 'feelings' diary, which I did. At first it was hard to know how I really did feel, but over the months, as I started to write, it just all flowed out of me – how I felt unwanted as a child, how I used to resent my husband and children and colleagues at work. I felt purged, really cleansed, and I was able to cry for the first time in years. I'm now so much happier and I have incredible energy – not just because I gave up working full-time, but because yoga helped me to release all the emotional tension I had held on to for years.

Exercises to Balance the Heart Chakra

YOGA POSTURES

Any posture that helps open up the chest area is beneficial for the Heart Chakra. Backward bends are therefore very good. Try the Cobra, where the hand position is near your chest. Also try the Fish and the Head of a Cow.

OTHER WAYS

Whenever possible, try surrounding yourself with nature. The greenness in nature is very therapeutic and will help to lift your energies. Try walking barefoot on the grass. Also touch and cuddle your loved ones as much as you can. Yoga helps you to tune in to your Heart Chakra and get in touch with your feelings.

Try closing your eyes and repeating the mantra 'My heart beats quietly and regularly with love'.

The Throat Chakra

- At the physical level, your Throat Chakra is related to your thyroid gland, vocal cords, ears and the endocrine system. Breathing problems, such as hyperventilation, asthma, emphysema and bronchitis, may indicate that your Throat Chakra is unbalanced. Other clues that this chakra needs working on include hypothyroidism, throat problems in general, mouth ulcers and hearing problems.
- The Throat Chakra is represented by the colour blue.
- This chakra is particularly concerned with how you communicate and express yourself in the world. A balanced Throat Chakra will help you put forward your feelings and ideas, and this in turn can lead to an understanding of your true path in life.
- If your Throat Chakra is blocked, you may find you have problems with words. People who speak very quietly or who are inarticulate may have a blocked Throat Chakra. If you suspect that you come across as cynical, hostile or sarcastic, this is another sign that you need to work on your Throat Chakra. If you do sometimes express yourself in a negative way, it is probably true to say that you are hiding your real self, partly because you lack confidence. In other words, this chakra may be blocked because, at another level, you are covering up with a false identity. This will make you very fatigued, even if you are unaware of this at a conscious level; trying to be someone you are not is very tiring. Remember, too, that how you verbalise your ideas and feelings helps to create your own reality - but negativity can actually create fatigue!
- If your Throat Chakra is too open, you may be over-talkative without being truly analytical, and you may dominate conversations without saying anything of value. Again, this is very exhausting, both for you and for others. Talking too much can be a defence mechanism that helps you avoid looking inwards and instead fills your life with trivia.
- If your Throat Chakra is balanced, you'll be able to interact with the world by talking, listening and reading - all of which help you to learn and express your true feelings clearly. If you are true to yourself and communicate your thoughts positively, you will start to realise and experience real energy - or prana.

Exercises to Balance the Throat Chakra

YOGA POSTURES

The Shoulder Stand, the Plough, the Bridge and the Fish are all excellent postures for energising the Throat Chakra.

OTHER WAYS

Singing and chanting are all beneficial therapies for the Throat Chakra. Chanting can heighten your awareness, aid meditation and help to balance your higher chakras. The vibration of sound will help you to tune in to your true self and will really aid your fight against fatigue. You can also try using the mantra Om, which I will explain at the end of this chapter.

Also, try keeping a feelings diary or writing poetry, reading, painting or learning a new skill. Practising pranayama or yoga breathing techniques is vital for all chakras, but has particular relevance for the Throat Chakra.

The Brow Chakra

- The Brow Chakra relates to your eyes, lower brain and nervous system (including the pituitary and pineal glands that are relevant for your hormones and are so often associated with fatigue, particularly if you are under stress). Your Brow Chakra is also responsible for your hypothalamus, often known as the Master Gland because it controls so many functions, including sleep, temperature regulation and your emotions. The hypothalamus is often implicated in cases of Chronic Fatigue Syndrome, because if it is not functioning properly your general vitality and emotional wellbeing will be affected.
- This chakra is symbolised by the colour indigo blue.
- Your Brow Chakra is responsible for your imagination and concentration. As one of your higher chakras, it is also related to your finer emotions and spiritual status.
- If this chakra is blocked, you may suffer from negative thoughts, learning difficulties, poor concentration, headaches and mental fatigue. In extreme cases, this can lead to confused thinking or even psychosis – a lack of understanding between reality and fantasy.

- If this chakra is too open too soon, you may have anxiety about your spiritual progress – especially if you are not sufficiently grounded by your Root Chakra or centred by your Solar Plexus Chakra.
- When the Brow Chakra is balanced, your creative spirit will flow freely. Your Brow Chakra is about using your intuition and creative force. Activation of this chakra also helps with visualisation, which in effect is seeing with the mind's eye. Visualisation is very useful as an aid to meditation, and a powerful tool for beating exhaustion.

Exercises to Balance the Brow Chakra

VISUALISATION

This exercise, called Candle Gazing, is commonly used in yoga to aid concentration for those who are new to meditation. It is easy to do and very effective.

First, light a candle in a darkened room. Sit a few feet away – on the floor or on a chair – and look at the flame. Try to clear your mind of everything else. After a few minutes, close your eyes. You will find that you can still see the candle flame, even though your eyes are closed. This is called the negative afterimage. Concentrate on this negative image of the flame. Try to keep your mind empty of everything but this image. When the image starts to fade, open your eyes and look at the candle again. Practise this with your eyes open and then closed for about five minutes, increasing the time as you become more comfortable with the meditation.

Think about how this exercise makes you feel. Notice any changes that happen as you practise this over the months.

YOGA POSTURES

The Pose of a Child and the Standing Dog Stretch are excellent for the Brow Chakra.

OTHER WAYS

If you suffer from mental fatigue, try visualisation, meditation and yoga breathing exercises. After practising any of the suggested exercises, always make sure you ground yourself with your Root Chakra by wriggling the base of your spine on the ground to connect yourself with the earth.

The Alternate Nostril breath, described in Chapter 4, is excellent for the Brow Chakra.

The Crown Chakra

- At the physical level, the Crown Chakra is responsible for your upper brain and, like the Brow Chakra, for your pituitary and pineal glands.
- It is represented by the colour violet, and also white, which is the whole colour spectrum. The Crown Chakra is an amalgamation of all the other chakras; if all the chakras are notes of a tune, the Crown Chakra can be said to be the whole melody.
- If your Crown Chakra is blocked, you may suffer from depression, and you may find it difficult to accept life as it is. You may feel imprisoned in your body, with no spiritual connection or direction from within. This will make you feel drained and exhausted.
- Conversely, if your Crown Chakra is too open, you may become too stuck in the spiritual world and be unable to relate to the real, physical here and now. This can bring about anxiety and fear.
- The Crown Chakra, if balanced, is about acceptance and peace as opposed to fear and despair. Because the Crown Chakra represents all our chakras together, it is concerned with understanding the total pattern of life and why we are here. As I have explained, yoga is about union, which includes the coming together of mind, body and spirit with the universe. If you truly want to beat fatigue, then you have to pay attention to your spiritual self as well as your physical body.

Exercises to Balance the Crown Chakra

You can balance this chakra best through a disciplined practice of meditation. This will free you from the constant mental exhaustion which results from the hum of thinking in your head. Meditation helps to enhance the slower Alpha waves of your brain, and to harmonise the hypothalamus and endocrine system, all of which affect your energy levels; so at this level it can be seen that meditation is essential for increasing vitality.

VISUALISATIONS

1 Close your eyes and relax as much as possible. Now imagine that you are breathing in a beautiful, translucent violet light at the point between your eyebrows. As you breathe out, this becomes a white light, which you breathe out through your Crown Chakra, up to the sky. Practise this for a few minutes.
2 Shut your eyes and imagine above your head a closed up lotus flower with many petals – as many as one thousand. The petals slowly start to open and, as they do, sunlight streams down into your head. Imagine this light and energy going through your head and down through all your chakras, slowly filling them with light.

YOGA POSTURES

The Pose of a Rabbit or Hare is a good posture for the Crown Chakra. (Experienced yoga students can practise the Head Stand every day; I have not covered this posture in this book as it is best learnt under supervision.)

Exercises to Balance All Your Chakras

Although you can work on each chakra individually, it is also important to work on all of them together so that you can achieve real balance and bring health and vitality into your life. The following exercise will help you to do this.

Visualisation

Sit on the floor with your legs crossed, or on the back of your heels if this is more comfortable. Sit upright and don't allow yourself to droop or sink into your hips. Keep your shoulders relaxed and down. Now imagine that the base of your spine has roots that go down through the floor into the ground, and that your head and the top of your spine are reaching upwards, into the sky. Only imagine this; although you are sitting upright your spine should be relaxed, not pulled. Now close your eyes. Breathe in then out, slowly, from your diaphragm. On the out-breath, imagine your breath going from the top of your head, down your spine and out into the ground. On the in-breath, breathe up through the base of your spine into the top of your head and out to the sky. Continue with this visualisation, with your breath going up your spine on the in-breath and down on the out-breath. Always ground yourself by ending on an out-breath. Practise this for three minutes, or longer if you feel comfortable.

Sound can be used for healing. Vibration, or sound, is energy and underlines everything in the universe. Because sound is energy, each word we use also has its own power. Chanting mantras are said to open our hearts and make love flow, as well as purifying the atmosphere around us. Chanting, also known as nada yoga, is said to be a direct way to connect with the higher self, or universal life force – as when we chant, the mind becomes still and we become very connected in the present moment.

Chanting with the Om Breath

Om is one of the best mantras to start with. It is said to incorporate all the vibrations of the universe and can help to balance and invigorate all the chakras and raise energy and healing as the vibrations stimulate the nerve endings. If practised every day, it can help you to tune in to your real self, thereby bringing about quite profound changes. It is also very relaxing, especially if you focus on the stillness between each breath. First, sit comfortably upright with the spine erect. Close your eyes, breathe in deeply from your diaphragm, open your mouth as wide as you can and as you breathe out sing 'aaaah' (as you do if a doctor is looking down your throat!). The sound is coming from the back of the throat.

Using the same out-breath, start to bring your mouth in to an 'o' shape so that the sound becomes 'ooohh'. You will feel the breath rise up to the top of the chest and the sound is coming out more from the front of the mouth. Finally, still breathing out, bring your lips together so that for the final part of the breath you are humming 'mmmm'.

When you put the sequence together on one out-breath, you should be humming an 'ah-oo-mm' sound (Om). Take a deep breath and repeat at least five times. When you have finished, let the silence wash over you, keeping your eyes closed for a couple of minutes.

the **secret** of **energy control** 4

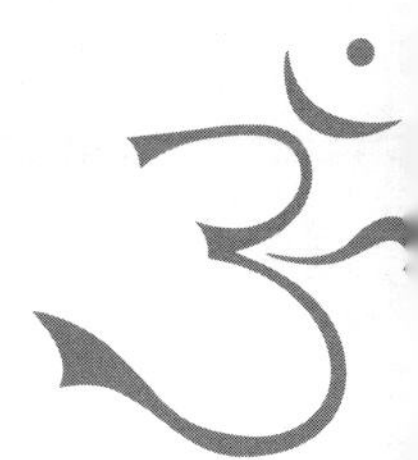

In the last chapter we looked at prana, the vital energy of the universe. In this chapter I will introduce you to pranayama, which will help you to control, store and direct this energy. If you practise the exercises given in this chapter, you will increase your vitality enormously.

Pranayama – Yoga Breathing Exercises

Prana can be controlled by using various yoga exercises, including the postures. However, one of the main ways to control it is to practise yoga breathing techniques, especially when combined with bandhas, which I will explain later. By controlling your breath you can help to control prana, and by learning to control this Universal Energy you can start to control your mind. This is possible because breathing helps to bring the mind under control; and because your emotions actually affect your breathing, you can therefore affect your emotional state by thinking about the way you breathe – and changing it! For example, if you are anxious or fearful, you breathe rapidly from your upper chest. This goes back to the 'fight or flight' syndrome that we looked at earlier. If you are really concentrating on something, you may notice that your breathing rate drops, or you may even hold your breath. If you are relaxed, your breathing becomes slow and deep. So next time you are in a stressful situation, try to slow down your breathing rate and see what difference it makes. A calm mind leads to a healthy body.

Before we go on to the pranayama exercises, it is important that you get your normal breathing rate under control. Make sure you are using your diaphragm and not breathing too rapidly. In Chapter 2 I asked you to lie down and isolate your ribs, then showed you how to use this area for breathing. Now I'd like you to try this again, but this time sitting upright in a chair; keeping your back straight. Put your hands around your ribcage so that your thumbs are pointing towards your back. This will help you feel the dome-shaped muscle of your diaphragm. Firstly, try to listen to your breathing and slow it down. Now balance it to an in-and-out rhythm. As you inhale, allow your ribcage to expand upwards, sideways, and into your back. As you slowly exhale, your hands should come closer together – you can gently squeeze your ribs together if you want to help this action. As your lower ribs move up and out with your in-breath, your diaphragm drops and stretches. When you breathe out, your diaphragm rises into a cone shape. Try breathing in through your nose for a count of four, and out for a count of four. This is one round.

What you are aiming to do is to breathe rhythmically, from your ribcage area, and to breathe no more than 10-12 rounds a minute. By doing this you are not over-breathing and you are using your diaphragm. This should influence your normal way of breathing, so do check yourself during the day to ensure that you are breathing more slowly and from your diaphragm, especially if you are in a stressful situation.

When you breathe in this way, your upper chest area may rise slightly, which is fine as long as you are not breathing just from this area. Incidentally, some yoga experts used to teach diaphragmatic breathing by getting students to breathe into their navel area, using a technique called the three-part or full breath. Nowadays however, it is generally accepted to be better practice – and more effective for energy production – to use the ribcage area just above the navel. Your abdomen should remain firm.

General Guidelines

Now that you have learned to breathe properly you are ready to learn the pranayama exercises, which I have divided into two sections. The first includes some basic routines which you can practise every day for about three months. Start with one or two every day, including perhaps the Kapalabhati Breath, which needs to be built up slowly. For the Alternate Nostril sequence, start with about one minute of practice and gradually increase to a maximum of 10.

When you feel happy that you are benefiting from these basic sequences, you can move on to the breath-retention exercises. Eventually, you can increase your pranayama practice from 10 up to a maximum of 20 minutes a day, choosing exercises that suit you from the selection I suggest. However, I would recommend that you do this only after lots of practice.

If you can persuade someone to read these instructions to you as you do the exercises, all the better; otherwise, read the exercises slowly and I can assure you that you will soon get the idea.

Before you start pranayama, bear in mind the following points:

- Your breathing should be rhythmic and smooth, not forced or jerky. Keep it slow.
- How you think is absolutely vital. The movement of your mind affects prana, so you should always think positively, imagining prana or energy filling your body as you practise. When you are doing the exercises, concentrate only on your breathing, the rhythm, and the idea of prana. Try not to let your mind wander. Keep your eyes closed, this will help your concentration. All these exercises are healing because they awaken prana, helping your whole system to become more balanced.
- Everything in the universe is vibration or energy – and in all vibration there is rhythm. So try to pay attention to the rhythm of your breathing.
- Practise pranayama after your yoga postures, not before – and always on an empty stomach. In the morning before breakfast is a good time. When you've finished, lie down in the Pose of Complete Rest for about five minutes.
- Always practise with an upright spine. This keeps the main nadi or energy channel open and thus helps the flow of prana.
- Always breathe through your nose unless otherwise instructed. The hairs in your nostrils help to filter out impurities, germs, dust and pollution. Breathing through your nose also warms the air which protects your lungs.
- Unless otherwise instructed, remember to keep your abdomen firm and don't allow it to balloon out. Firm means controlled – not rigid.
- A cycle consists of one inhalation and exhalation – with retention if indicated.

- If you feel tired or dizzy, stop! Check with your doctor first if you are suffering from heart or lung problems. Never strain and never try to hold your breath for too long.
- Always exhale first so that you start a round on an in-breath.
- And finally, if you feel any stress during the day, practise some pranayama exercises and visualise that you are breathing in peace and strength and breathing out negativity. You will be amazed at how effective this is!

Basic Pranayama Exercises

Kapalabhati

This is an excellent exercise to use at the beginning of pranayama because it cleanses the lungs and prepares them for the exercises to follow. It is incredibly invigorating and involves a dynamic out-breath in short bursts, followed by a slower inhalation. As long as you return to normal breathing afterwards, you will receive enormous benefit from Kapalabhati. This breath removes stale air from your lungs and brings about a rapid expulsion of carbon dioxide so that your blood becomes saturated with oxygen. This stimulates cellular (internal) breathing, which is particularly beneficial if you lead a sedentary life. Kapalabhati breathing will calm your nervous system, massage your digestive tract and, most importantly, literally 'irrigate' your brain! Your brain will be filled with fresh blood which will stimulate the endocrine, pituitary and pineal glands. In this way the brain is washed in oxygen-rich blood and cleansed of stagnant or sluggish circulating blood. Poor blood flow to the brain has been shown to be evident in cases of Chronic Fatigue Syndrome, so you can see why the Kapalabhati breathing is so incredibly energising.

A word of caution - do not practise this exercise if you have serious eye or ear complaints, if you suffer from high or low blood pressure, a hiatus hernia, any lung disorder, or if you are pregnant. Build up this sequence slowly from one round of 10 breaths to a maximum of 120 breaths, or 10 rounds of 10 fast breaths, which would eventually be done in one minute. I would suggest you add a round of 10 breaths each week, going from 10 to 20, then 30, and so on until you reach 120.

Kapalabhati is very energising, which is why I am including it here. But I have to add that it is best practised under supervision, so if you know of a friendly yoga teacher, you may like to ask for some help.

METHOD

Sit with your spine upright and identify your diaphragm area around your lower ribcage, as before. Now, using your abdomen like a piston, contract the muscles sharply to cause a violent expulsion of air – as if someone has punched you. Next, you will have to breathe in to fill the vacuum created by your out-breath. This should be automatic – rather like sneezing with your mouth closed! Repeat this exercise rapidly for 10 breaths. This is one round of Kapalabhati. Relax for three breaths. In your second week of practice, add 10 more breaths (another round), then rest again. Gradually build up to 120 breaths a minute, as explained above. Remember; this exercise should not be practised for more than a minute in any one session.

If you are feeling tired during the day, try practising Kapalabhati. It really does combat fatigue and drowsiness because toxins are dissolved and the brain is recharged. This breath also increases concentration, improves memory and stimulates the intellect. It is especially refreshing if you have been working at a computer or in an office. Because this is technically a hyperventilation exercise (in other words, it induces a rapid intake of oxygen), remember to return to normal breathing when you have finished, so you do not wash out too much carbon dioxide.

Alternate Nostril Breathing

You may remember I explained that your body has three main nadis that help conduct your prana or life energy throughout the body. Two of these are located in the nostrils and are related to positive and negative energies. This means that in order to be healthy, these nadis need to be kept clear and in balance. Alternate nostril breathing helps to clear these two main nadis and also encourages harmony between the left and right sides of the brain. Science now tells us that we use one side of our brain more than the other. For example, creative people such as artists tend to use the right side, whereas scientists and mathematicians favour their left side, which is used for more rational and logical thinking. Using alternate nostril breathing can help to balance both hemispheres of the brain.

METHOD

Curl the index and middle finger into the palm of your right hand, so that you can use your thumb to block one nostril and your ring finger the other. Support your elbow with your other hand if necessary. If you get tired, swap hands. Start by exhaling through both nostrils. Then block your right nostril and inhale through the left to a slow count of four. Now block your left nostril and exhale through the right using the same rhythm of four. Then inhale through your right nostril, block it, and exhale through your left. This completes one round. Continue like this, concentrating on the rhythm and making sure that both the in- and out-breath are complete and even. Practise this for one minute to start with, then increase the time. Close your eyes to aid concentration.

The Ha Breath

This breath uses a sweeping arm movement which helps to pump great energy into your body. It also helps to cleanse stale air from your lungs.

METHOD

Stand upright, keeping your spine straight. Breathe out. Now breathe in and lift your arms up over your head. Breathe out. Breathe in, bending your knees and taking your arms slightly behind your head. Now, as you breathe out, let your trunk flop forwards, bend your knees, let your arms swing in front of you and open your mouth and force the air out. As you do so say 'haaaa', sighing the air out. This out-breath should last for about five seconds. Hold your position, relaxing your arms, head and trunk down for a few seconds, and then repeat five times. Keep the knees slightly bent as you relax down to protect the back.

Traditional Yoga Breathing

This exercise is very calming, and simple to do.

METHOD

Breathe in slowly for a count of four, then breathe out slowly for a count of six. You can vary this rhythm to suit your natural breathing pattern – for example, you may like to breathe in for a count of six and out for a count of eight. Extending the exhalation calms down the central nervous system and is very good to do if you feel stressed.

This completes the basic pranayama exercises, which you should practise every day for about three months. Then you can move on to the more advanced breath-retention exercises. But first I will explain bandhas.

Bandhas

Bandhas are locks that you can use to increase the effectiveness of your breath-retention exercises, because they help to seal in energy or prana. Bandha is a Sanskrit word meaning to tie, control or lock, and the positions involve various muscular contractions which affect the circulation of your blood, your nerves and endocrine system. There are three main bandhas: the Chin Lock, the Abdomen Lock, and the Root Lock. I'm going to describe these exercises here so that you can try them. When you feel comfortable with them, you can use them where indicated in the next sequence of pranayama.

The Chin Lock

This position compresses and stimulates the thyroid gland. It does this so effectively that you must not use it if you have an overactive thyroid. It is very beneficial if you are suffering from fatigue.

Inhale, then, holding your breath, press your chin down firmly into your chest, between the collarbones. As you exhale, slowly lift your chin back to its normal position.

The Abdomen Lock

Inhale, then exhale and pull the abdomen up and back towards the spine. Then breathe normally as you hold.

The Root Lock

This lock involves contracting your anal sphincter muscles. It tones up the lower bowel and pelvic floor area, prevents constipation and haemorrhoids and is good for balancing your Root Chakra.

Inhale, hold your breath and contract your anus and pelvic floor muscles. Exhale and relax. Repeat twice. As you do this, focus your attention on the anus as you contract it, then imagine the point above this and contract that too. The Root and Abdomen Lock are sometimes held in a yoga sequence to increase stability in the postures.

Combined Lock

To combine these three locks, stand upright, breathe in and lower your chin to your chest. Hold your breath and pull the lower abdominal area up towards your spine and pull up your anal muscles. Breathe out slowly and release the locks.

The following sequences – which involve all the bandhas – are excellent for increasing energy.

Imaginary Rowing

Sit on the floor, with your legs out straight. Now imagine that you are pulling on the oars of a boat. Lean forward, arms outstretched and exhale. As you start to inhale, pull on the imaginary oars as you start to lean back, pressing your chin into your chest and tightening your abdominal, pelvic floor and anal muscles. Hold your breath then release, rowing forward as you breathe out. Repeat this sequence up to 10 times.

Pot Stirring

For a variation on the above, pretend you are stirring a giant pot. From the same position, hold your hands together with your arms outstretched. Now move your arms in a large circle in time with your breath. At the end of your in-breath, your chin should be on your chest, with your pelvic floor, anal and abdominal muscles tight. At the end of the out-breath, you should be leaning forward, outstretched over your legs.

Mudras

As well as bandhas, there are also mudras – hand positions that help close the circuits of energy in your body and direct the breath. You may like to use a basic position known as jnana mudra when you are practising the next sequence of pranayama exercises. It is very simple – just touch the tip of your index finger with the tip of your thumb, then either rest your hands on your knees (palms up), or keep the rest of your fingers outstretched. As well as closing your energy circuit, this mudra is said to stop the energy leaking out of your extremities.

Breath-retention Exercises

In yoga, it is thought that we are allocated a set number of breaths, so that life is measured in breaths rather than years. Therefore, it is thought that slowing down your breath will help to increase your life span. In pranayama, as well as learning to slow down your breathing, you can learn to hold or retain your breath. This can greatly increase your energy because your respiration affects the circulation of your blood and is a powerful tonic for the whole system. Holding your breath helps prana to flow because it stimulates cellular breathing by helping your cells to absorb oxygen and to evacuate carbon dioxide more effectively. In other words, it gives a better 'digestion' of inhaled air. Breath retention also stimulates the spleen and makes it expel large quantities of red corpuscles into the bloodstream. It also produces heat in your body and can even increase the activity of your brain, because fluids are circulated more efficiently. They are contra-indicated, however, if you have high blood pressure or heart conditions.

I am now going to describe seven different breath-retention exercises. Start by selecting a few every day and gradually build up to about 10 minutes' practice. You will further increase your energy if you use the bandhas. As a guide, I suggest you use the Chin Lock when holding your breath after an inhalation, and the Abdomen and Root Locks when holding your breath after an exhalation, unless otherwise instructed.

1 To start with, take five ordinary in-and-out-breaths, then hold the last one for a few seconds, holding then releasing the Chin Lock. Listen in to your body as you do so. Then exhale slowly and smoothly, pushing the air out by contracting your ribcage muscles. Don't breathe out suddenly. In this way you are controlling the inhalation, retention and exhalation. Practise a round of six per session.

2 The next exercise combines breath retention with alternate nostril breathing. Using the hand positions I described, block your right nostril and exhale slowly through your left nostril for a count of four seconds. Inhale through the left nostril then hold your breath for four seconds by blocking both nostrils; finally exhale through your right nostril for four seconds. Now do the whole exercise the other way round – inhaling through your right nostril, blocking both nostrils and holding your breath, then releasing and exhaling through your left nostril. This completes one round. I suggest you do six rounds, then increase if you would like to.

3 For a more advanced version of the above exercise, add a visualisation to increase the prana that is absorbed. Inhale through your left nostril for a count of four, then close both nostrils and retain the breath for a count of four. Then breathe out through your right nostril for a count of six. To complete the round, breathe in through your right nostril for a count of four, block your nostrils and hold the breath for a count of four, then breathe out slowly through your left nostril for a count of six. Use the Chin Lock when you are holding your breath. Do this exercise only if you can do so without straining. As you are holding your breath, imagine that you are sending a current of prana down your spine, through your chakras into your Root Chakra. Remember to keep your breath slow and smooth.

4 Breathe in through both nostrils for a count of two. Hold for a count of four using the Chin Lock, then breathe out for a count of four, releasing the Chin Lock. As you do this, imagine that you are absorbing prana as pure energy into your whole body. You might like to think of this as a colour. By using your mind in this way, you are increasing the absorption and circulation of prana. When you use the Chin Lock while you are holding your breath, close your eyes and think about the energy you are storing in your solar plexus. As you breathe out, imagine that the current of prana is spreading from your Solar Plexus Chakra to the rest of your body: to every organ, muscle, cell and nerve. Pay special attention to sending prana to your head and think about how it is invigorating and stimulating

you. If you have any area you wish to heal, you can send the prana there. Repeat this several times. Really concentrate on this exercise, thinking only of your breath and prana.

5 The first four exercises involve holding the breath after the inhalation. In this one you retain the breath after your exhalation, using a breathing pattern called the Square, because of its 4:4:4:4 pattern. Breathe in for a count of four, hold your breath for a count of four, breathe out for four and then hold your breath for another count of four before you start the round again. You can vary this pattern if you like – for example, you can use 6:6:6:6. In addition, you could use the Chin Lock after the inhalation, and the Abdomen and Root Lock when you are holding your breath after the exhalation. You could also try using this square rhythm when you are out walking, using your steps to count. The rhythm here is most important as it prepares you for withdrawing the senses, ready for meditation. Practise a few rounds to start with and increase up to 30.

6 This exercise helps to dispel toxins from the skin by generating heat in the body – you may find that it makes you perspire! Exhale, then inhale slowly for a count of four. Hold your breath for four. Then inhale again for a count of four. Hold the breath again for a count of four, then inhale and hold for another count of four. Exhale very slowly. Do two more rounds of this, then relax.

7 Lie on your back on the floor, or on your bed. Close your eyes and visualise a ball of white healing light above the crown of your head. Use the rhythm 8:4:8:4. As you inhale for a count of eight, feel light coming up through the soles of your feet, passing through your chakras and revitalising your body, until it meets a ball of white light at the Crown Chakra. Hold your breath for four, then exhale and move the light from the top of your head back down to your feet. Hold your breath. When you start the next round of breathing, use the rhythm to slowly circle the light around your body, from your feet to your head and back again, so that you are surrounded in an egg of white, healing light. This exercise can make you feel really calm, yet at the same time energised and strong.

The last few exercises are used as a preparation for meditation. If you spend a few months practising pranayama, you will become much calmer and find your concentration improves. In Chapter 11 we will look at meditation in more detail.

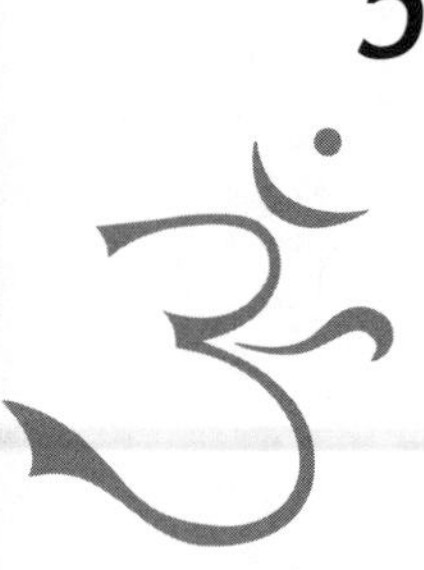

the **postures** – getting started

In the next four chapters I shall be covering all the postures in yoga that will help you beat fatigue.

Basic Guidelines

1 It is very important to remember that yoga is non-competitive, so work at your own pace without pushing or straining. Be comfortable and relax into the postures.

2 Always start with a relaxation posture. Then do some short warm-up stretches. Relax between each posture. And always finish with a relaxation posture such as the Pose of Complete Rest. If you want to beat fatigue, there are three important things to learn - relaxation, relaxation and more relaxation! This is not the same as stretching out in front of the TV, but a conscious letting go of muscle tension. I put a lot of emphasis on relaxation as it is something we don't do often enough, and as I explained in Chapter 1 when I talked about stress, tension is a major cause of fatigue. So don't feel guilty - relaxation postures are as important as 'active' postures in yoga. And anyway, yoga is about being, not doing!

3 Try to think of each posture as an exercise in meditation. By this I mean that you should become completely involved and concentrate only on the posture so that your mind doesn't wander. Think about the flow of energy as you breathe. Above all, enjoy your yoga practice - think of it as your treat, your time, not just something else on a long list of things that you have to do. Keep your mind in the here and now during your practice.

4 Breathe through your nose as you work. Remember to breathe normally when you hold a posture. In yoga, you work in rhythm with your breath. I'll explain this as we go along, but as a rough rule of thumb, you breathe in when you lift a limb, and out when you lower it.
5 Always come out of a posture very carefully, not suddenly or jerkily.
6 It is beneficial to repeat a posture two or three times, and to hold it for as long as you feel is right.
7 You must check with your doctor first if you have any health problems, including the following: heart trouble, high blood pressure, eye problems such as glaucoma, ear trouble or back problems. (Yoga can help with some back problems, but you need to check with your physiotherapist, chiropractor or osteopath about which exercises are relevant for you - some postures could make your condition worse.) If you are pregnant and haven't done yoga before, it's very important that you consult a yoga teacher, because some of the postures in this book should not be practised during pregnancy.
8 Do not eat for at least two hours before doing any yoga postures. This is because digestion uses up energy. Empty your bladder first. Wear loose, comfortable clothing such as leggings or tracksuit bottoms with a T-shirt or fleece. Ideally, you should work in bare feet as you are liable to slip when doing some of the standing postures. If your feet get cold you can wear socks with rubber grips. You may like to use a blanket for relaxation. Make sure you have enough space to work. Switch off the phone so that you won't be disturbed.
9 Do not do the inverted postures if you are menstruating or if you have high blood pressure. If you have asthma, be careful of inversions.
10 Always, always balance your postures. If you work on your right side, such as in the Triangle, you must work on your left side too. You must always counterpose - for example, if you do some backward bends, you then need to do some forward bends. As you do more yoga, your body will know when to counterpose; it will start to feel its natural balance so that you will know you need to bend forward after you have been bending backwards.
11 Try to practise for a minimum of 20 minutes a day. A full yoga session usually lasts 90 minutes. At home, if you can do one hour once a day, that is brilliant. You will see results faster. However; 20 minutes is better than no minutes, and twice a week is better than not at all. Aim to get into a regular routine, perhaps setting your alarm clock earlier and doing your yoga practice first thing in the morning.

12 If you have Chronic Fatigue Syndrome, start very slowly and listen to your body all the time. See Chapters 9 and 10 for yoga routines especially designed for CFS sufferers. However; all the postures in this chapter are suitable for people with CFS, unless the illness is very severe.

In this book, as you will have realised, I emphasise prana and pranayama (Universal Energy, and control of this through breathing). All yoga postures are designed to direct prana or vital energy to different parts of the body, and each pose works on one or more of your energy centres or chakras. However; in order to maximise the use of prana, I would like you to approach these postures in a slightly different way. As you do your yoga poses in rhythm with your breathing, I want you to think about and visualise the energy running through your system.

When you do this you will see that visualisation and proper breath control help the flow of energy in your body. There is scientific evidence that visualizing, or thinking about a posture, increases its effect. Psychologists at Manchester Metropolitan University in the UK have discovered that those who think about doing an exercise can improve their muscle groups by up to an additional 16 per cent, providing they imagine the feeling of the response they would get if they were actually doing the exercise. This is because most of the areas in the brain related to physical movement don't know the difference between doing a task and imagining it! I'm not suggesting that you shouldn't actually do the postures, but I am making the point that if you visualise your yoga poses as you work on them you will have a powerful way of encouraging prana.

Finally, a reminder: doing these yoga postures will help your whole system and lead to better health and energy. You will breathe properly and your circulation, organs, muscles, skeleton, ligaments, joints, spine, digestion, endocrine and nervous system will all be helped. These postures will also help to purify your body by removing toxins, and will make your mind strong as you develop stability and concentration. Yoga will help to bring your body, mind and spirit into harmony – and, best of all, it really will beat fatigue!

Working out a Daily Routine

It's very simple. In the next four chapters you will find postures listed under the following headings: Relaxation Postures, Warm-up Exercises, Lying Down Poses, Sitting Postures, Backward Bends, Standing Postures, Twists, and Inverted Postures. Forward bends are included in the Sitting and Standing sections. All you have to do is choose one or two postures from each category to make up your own daily routine. Those marked with one star (*) are easier than those marked with two, so should be practised first before you move on. Try to vary the postures so that you don't do the same ones each time. As you feel stronger, you can add more postures from each category. Remember to start and finish a session with relaxation, and to do some warm-up stretches before the poses. As I mentioned, you always need to counter a forward- or backward-bending posture with one that takes you in the opposite direction. If you don't want to make up your own routine, I've included three daily sequences that you can use.

If you are new to yoga, start with the postures with one star. Only when you feel strong enough should you move on to the two-star postures. In yoga, the more advanced you become, the longer you will be able to hold a posture, so at the beginning, hold the posture just for a few seconds and build up your tolerance slowly. As a very rough guide, you will find that backward bends are energising and forward bends are calming. If you have CFS, stick to the postures marked with one star.

Tip

Before you start, you may find it helpful to record the exercise instructions slowly onto an audio tape so that you can carry out the poses without having to look at the book all the time. Or you might like to ask a friend to read them out to you.

Relaxation Postures

The Pose of Complete Rest *

This posture is also known as The Corpse, the literal translation from the Sanskrit. It is so called because when performed properly, both your body and mind should be completely still. We have already covered this posture in Chapter 2, but as it is so important, I would like to go over it once again. It is said that 20 minutes of relaxation is equivalent to five hours of sleep, so this really is an invaluable posture to practise. This is said to be the most difficult posture to master but the most important.

1 Lie down with your eyes closed. Cover yourself with a blanket if you are cold. Try to relax as much as possible. Let your legs flop apart and rotate slightly outwards. Your palms should be facing upwards, but only if this is comfortable. Some people like to put their hands on their abdomen instead.
2 Now go through each body part, first tensing then relaxing it. Start with your feet and progress up to your legs, hands, arms, neck, shoulders, back, abdomen area, torso, jaws, face, forehead, and the back of your head. Pay particular attention to your shoulders, neck, jaws and abdomen, the areas where most tension is stored. In fact, you might like to think of your abdominal area as the hub of a wheel, from where relaxation spreads to all the other parts. You can do this by imagining a soothing, yellow, warm colour expanding outwards from this area, sending relaxing waves to the rest of your body.
3 Really concentrate on each part as you go through the pose, and try not to let your mind wander. Let your breath flow naturally. As you relax, your breathing should become deeper and slower. Feel yourself sinking into your support. Let all tension flow away. Try and hold onto this feeling of being relaxed and carry it with you throughout the day, so that if you become tense, you can consciously relax again.

Quick Tension Reliever *

This is an excellent way to relax quickly if you haven't the time to go through the full relaxation sequence.

Lie on the floor. Breathe in and lift your head, legs and arms slightly up from the floor - no more than a few inches. Now, holding your breath, tighten everything as much as possible. Screw up your face, make fists with your hands, clench your buttocks and really grip everything as firmly as you can. Then breathe out with a big sigh - 'haaa' - and let everything flop back onto the floor. Repeat twice more.

Pigeon Hole Visualisation *

This is another relaxation that is excellent to use at the beginning of a yoga class or meditation practice, when your head may be buzzing from the outside world and all the things you have to do. It is also very good as an aid to concentration.

1 First, relax as much as you physically can. Close your eyes.
2 Now, think of all your problems and all the things you have to do. Examine everything that is cluttering up your mind. Imagine that in front of you is a large wooden pigeon-hole unit, like those that hold letters and keys behind the reception desk in a hotel. Now imagine all your problems and responsibilities flying into the pigeon holes. As they do so, a shutter comes down and, for now, your troubles have been put aside and you don't need to think about them. Your mind is clear.
3 If you want you can open just one shutter to concentrate on any task you are doing. (For example, if you are in the car, open the shutter called 'driving' so that you concentrate on that one task and nothing else.) For now, you need to open the shutter called 'yoga postures'.
4 Remind yourself that this is your time to practise yoga and that you can attend to other needs when you finish. For the duration of your session there is nothing to be done, solved or thought about that can't wait until the end of your yoga practice. Your mental pigeon hole has taken away all your thoughts and problems for now.

After your yoga session you can carry on using this mental image so that throughout the day you have just one shutter open related to every task you do. In this way you can focus on what you are doing without worrying about anything else.

The Windmill *

This isn't strictly a relaxation posture, but I've included it here because it is very soothing and excellent for breath control. You can do this sitting down if you prefer.

1 Stand upright, keeping your shoulders relaxed, with your arms by your side.
2 Now, on an in-breath, swing your arms together towards your abdomen, then lift them up over your head. On an out-breath, circle your arms outwards and down to your sides. Repeat up to five times.
3 Do this very slowly, making big, circling, sweeping movements with your arms.
4 Now change direction so that you are circling your arms the other way.

This exercise pumps air and prana into your body and so is also very energising.

The Pose of a Child *

This is an excellent pose to do between postures. If you have problems relaxing on your back, you may like to try this instead.

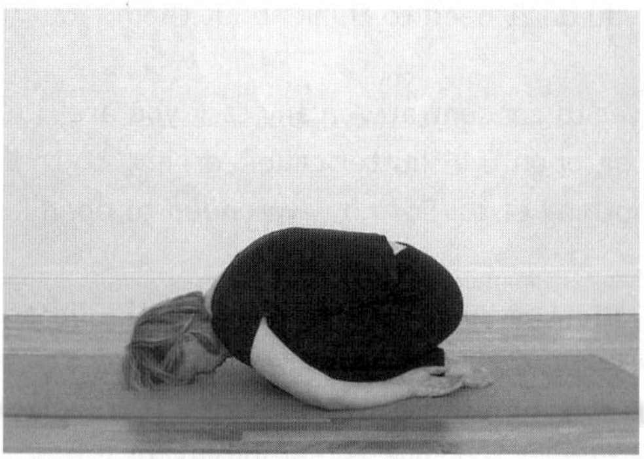

The Pose of a Child

1 Kneel, and sit up straight, without slumping, keeping your hips on your heels.
2 Now stretch forward and take your forehead down onto the floor. If you like, or if you have high blood pressure, you can rest your head on blocks or a book.
3 Take your arms to the side of your body, with your palms turned up, and relax.

This posture, with your head slightly lower than your heart, helps with blood flow to the brain so that your whole system is energised. As it is a forward bend, this posture can be used to counter a backward bend. If you have high blood pressure, put your head on a cushion.

Warm-up Exercises

Basic Stretching

*

You must always start your yoga practice with a few warm-up stretches so that you don't damage any of your muscles. You can do your stretches lying down or standing up, whichever you prefer.

LYING DOWN STRETCH

1 Lie down with your eyes closed.
2 Now, on an in-breath, slowly stretch your arms up over your head, stretching your hands away from your shoulders as much as you can. At the same time, stretch out your legs and point your toes. Pull your feet away from your hips. Hold for a few seconds.
3 On an out-breath, sigh 'haaa' and bring your arms back down to your sides and relax everything. Hold for a few seconds, then repeat the stretch twice more.

Incidentally, you sigh 'haaa' because it helps with the expulsion of old, stale air, and the intake of oxygen on the next breath.

STANDING STRETCHES

1 With your feet just a few inches apart, lift your arms over your head and press the palms of the hands together, stretching up towards the ceiling. Keep your hips straight and tilt the upper part of your body over to the right; opening your arms to parallel and stretch out. Come back to the centre and stretch up further.

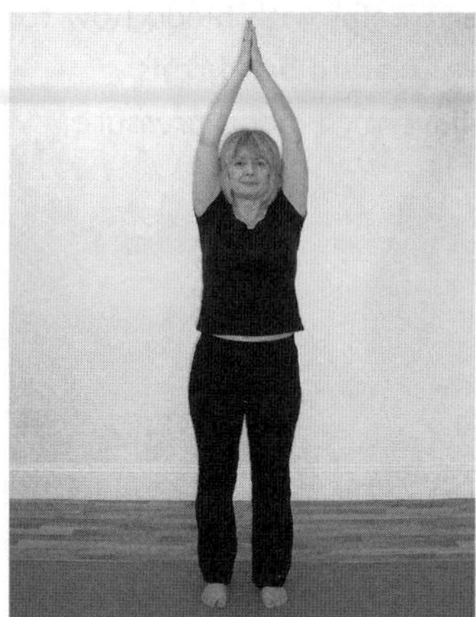

Arms raised over head

2 Now bend the upper half of your body slightly to the left and stretch. Then come back to the centre. Breathe in as you stretch up and out as you stretch to each side.

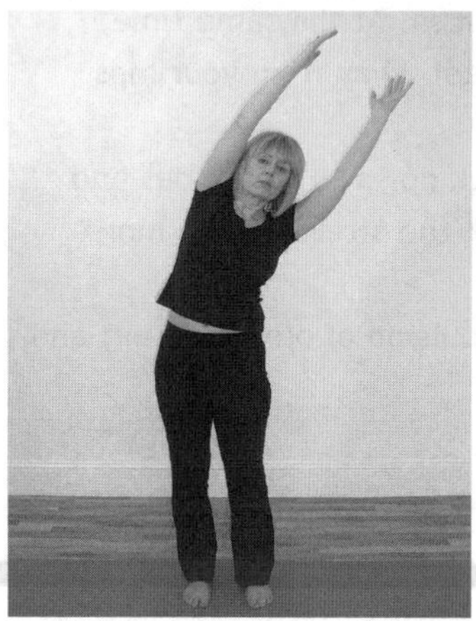

Upper half of body stretched

3 Now bend your trunk down and swing your arms towards your feet. If you can touch your toes do so, but only if you can do this without straining. Otherwise, bend your knees slightly so you can reach down.

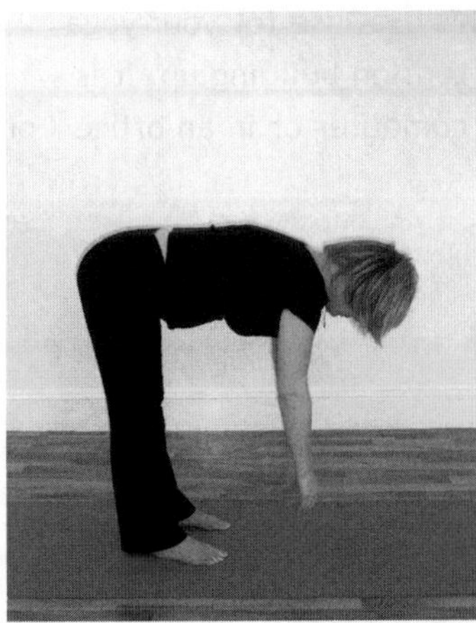

Moving into forward bend with back straight

4 To finish, come up slowly and put your hands on the back of your hips. Slowly lean back from your pelvis into a very gentle back bend but don't take the head too far back.

Neck Roll

*

We all carry a lot of tension in our neck and shoulders - often without realizing - and this can add to the picture of fatigue. As well as using this exercise for your yoga session, you may like to try it during the day if you feel tension building up. It is particularly good if you work sitting down - such as at a computer or in an office - or if you do a lot of driving.

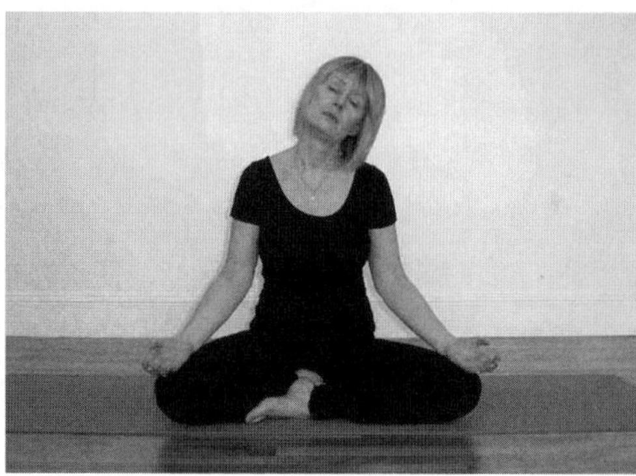

Neck roll to the right

1 Find a position that feels comfortable - sitting in a chair, kneeling, or sitting cross-legged. Keep upright, but relaxed.
2 Think about your spine. Is there any tension there? Let go of any tightness without slumping.
3 Think about how your head is positioned on your shoulders. Your head should not be hanging too far forward or straining too far back. Put your fingers on the back of your neck and work out how to hold your head in a way that causes the least tension in your neck. Your head should pivot freely on your atlas joint - where the skull meets the spine - and there should be no compression there. Think of a string coming out of the top of your head, lifting it up towards the ceiling.
4 On an out-breath, bring your chin slowly down towards your chest in time with your breath. On an in-breath, return it to the centre. On an out-breath, roll your head slightly back, keeping your jaw closed. Don't take it too far back. Breathe in and come back to the centre. Repeat this movement three times.

5 Now breathe in, and on the out-breath slowly roll your right ear towards your right shoulder. Breathe in again, and on the next two out-breaths see if you can take your ear a little further towards your shoulder. Pause, then on an in-breath bring your head back to the centre. On an out-breath, roll your left ear towards your left shoulder. Again, see if you can slowly take your ear a little further towards your shoulder on the next two out-breaths. On an in-breath, bring your head back to the centre. Repeat this three times.
6 Finally, still sitting upright and making sure you are not slumping, slowly look over your right shoulder on an out-breath. Return your head to the centre, then on the next out-breath gently take your head a little further to the right. Take your head back to the centre then repeat again. On the third out-breath, you should be able to take your head even further round to the right, but don't force it. Repeat on your left side, making sure that your trunk is facing forward and pressing down on the base of the spine to improve the flexibility in your neck.

Shoulder Shrug and Roll *

1 Sit or kneel as in the Neck Roll.
2 Now shrug your shoulders by putting them up towards your ears on the in-breath letting them flop down on the out-breath. Do this several times. Each time, as they relax down, they should come further away from your ears.

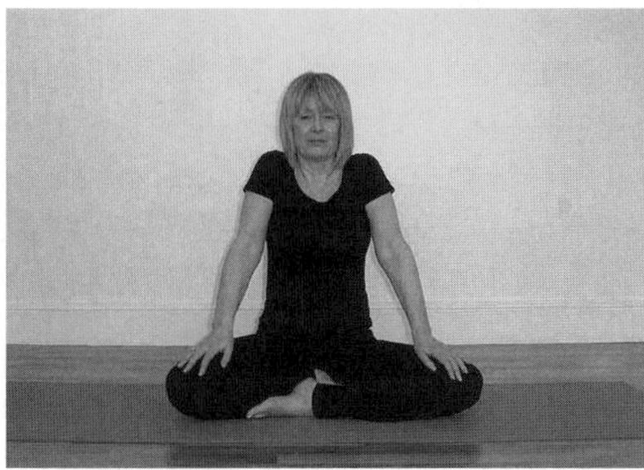

Shoulder shrug towards the ears

3 Now gently roll your shoulders in big circles, allowing your arms to flop as you do so. Do this several times, then circle your shoulders the other way. You can bend your arms and put your hands on your shoulders if you prefer. Keep the movements slow, in time with your breathing.

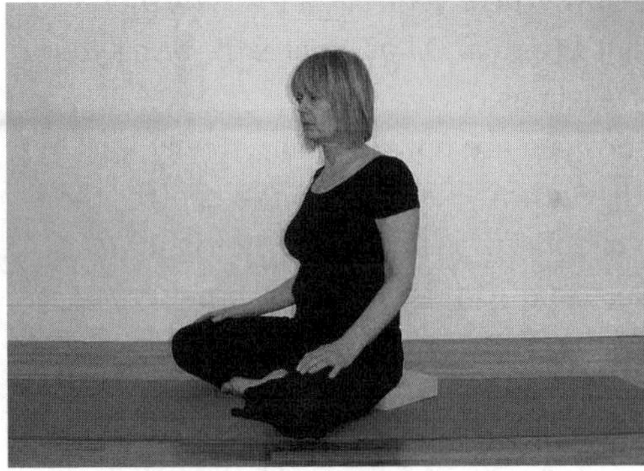

Shoulder roll to the back

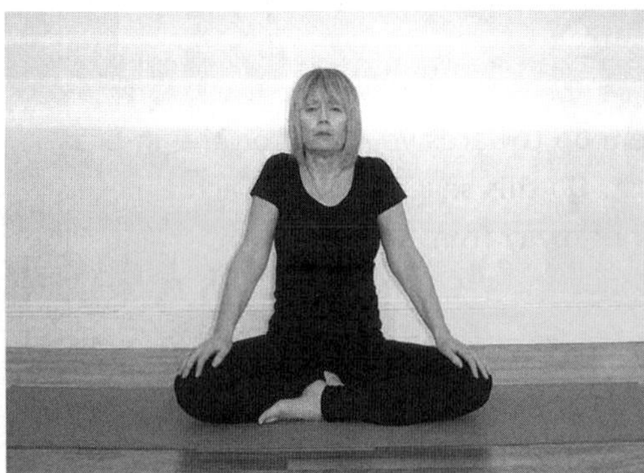

Shoulder roll to the front

Joint Exercises

The expression 'use it or lose it' is very apposite in relation to joints. These exercises will help to keep your joints supple and mobile so that if you practise them regularly, you shouldn't suffer from stiffness as you get older.

Elbows and Shoulders *

1 Sit in a comfortable position.
2 Now slowly circle your wrists about five times, then change direction.
3 Next, hold your arms out at shoulder level in an L-shape, with your elbows bent and your forearms pointing upwards. Push your hands back.
4 Now keep the upper part of your arm still as you bend your lower or forearms slowly until your hands point downwards. Your arms should still be in an L-shape. Push the palms of your hands back. Look at your upper arms to make sure they haven't dropped.

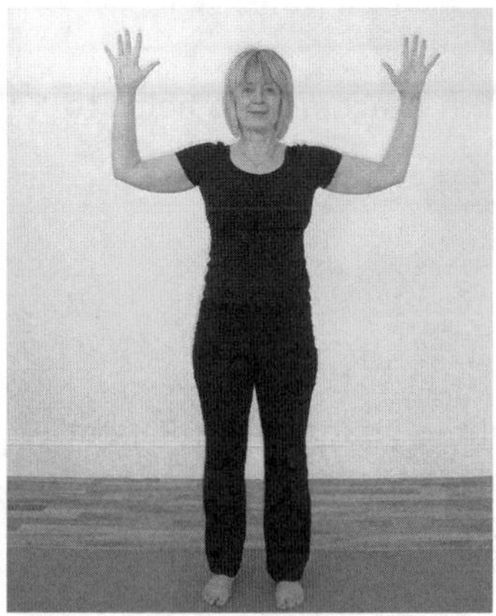

Arms in an L-shape

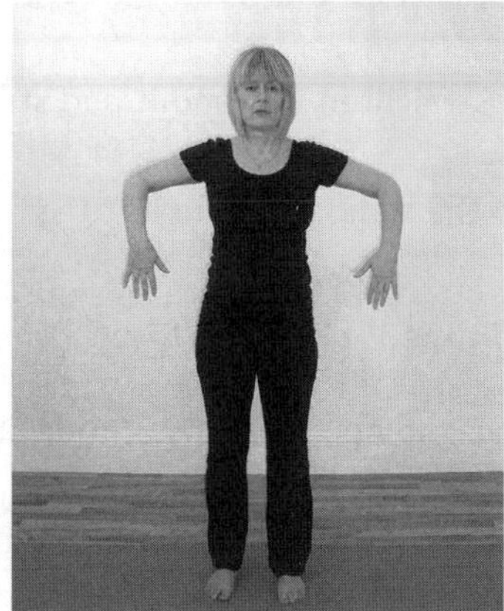

Hands pointing downwards

You will probably hear lots of creaks from your elbows and shoulders, which is a good sign! The tricky thing here is to keep your upper arms as still as possible, otherwise you are not mobilising your elbows enough. The picture shows this from a standing position but you can do this sitting.

Ankles *

1 Sit on a chair and cross one leg over the other.
2 Stretch your toes forward and back to get some movement in them. Now try and separate your toes, then give them a good wriggle.
3 Next, stretch your heels forward and pull your toes back.
4 Finally, circle your ankle slowly about five times one way, then five times the other way. Change legs.

Knees *

1 Still sitting on your chair; stretch your right leg out in a straight line and flex and point your toes.
2 Now bend your leg, straighten it, bend it and straighten it again. This helps to mobilise the knee.
3 Change over and do the same with the left leg.

Fingers *

1 To mobilise your finger joints, make fists, then straighten your fingers. Repeat several times.
2 Now wriggle your fingers as if you were playing the piano, or typing quite fast.
3 Finally, give your fingers a good shake.

Pelvic Lift

This is a good exercise for mobilising the pelvis, and one that will help you later when you are learning the Mountain Pose, which is about good posture. It is also beneficial for the pelvic floor muscles and the waist, and will help you in forward stretching postures.

1 Lie on the floor on your back with your legs bent at the knees, hip-width apart, with your ankles under your knees. You can put your hand on the abdomen to check the breath.

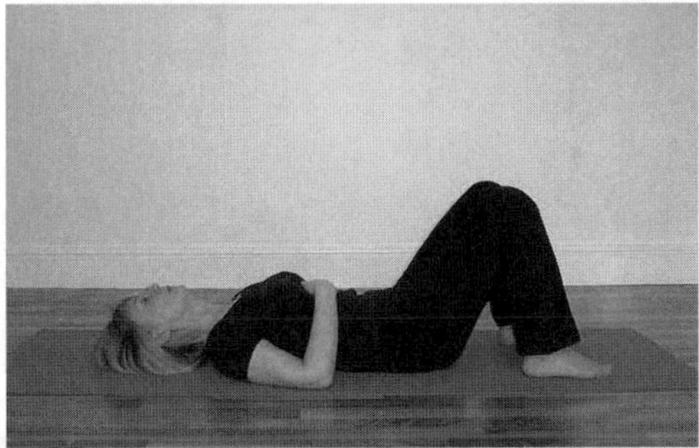

Pelvic Lift - start position

2 Relax, then on an out-breath start to press your waist into the floor. As you do so, your hips and pelvic area will start to rise slightly so that you are tilting your pelvis back; your hips should still be on the floor. Hold for a few seconds, tightening the abdominal muscles. Now on an in-breath, slowly roll the hips down and relax.

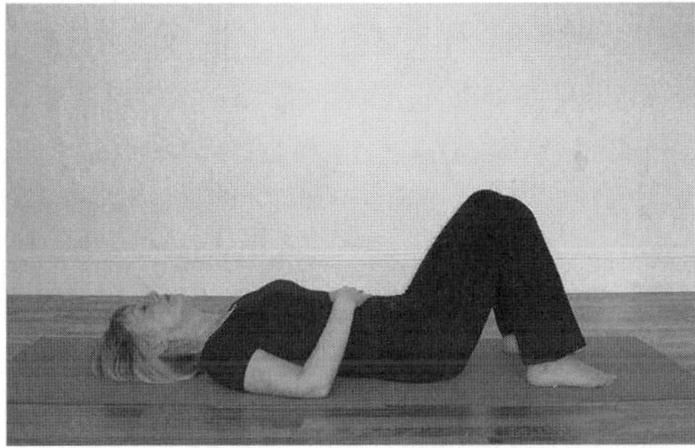

Pelvic Lift - tilted

3 When you have finished this pelvic movement, bring your knees to your chest and have a gentle rock from side to side. Then, with one hand on each knee and the knees together slowly circle your knees first one way, then the other. This gives a good massage to the back of the spine.

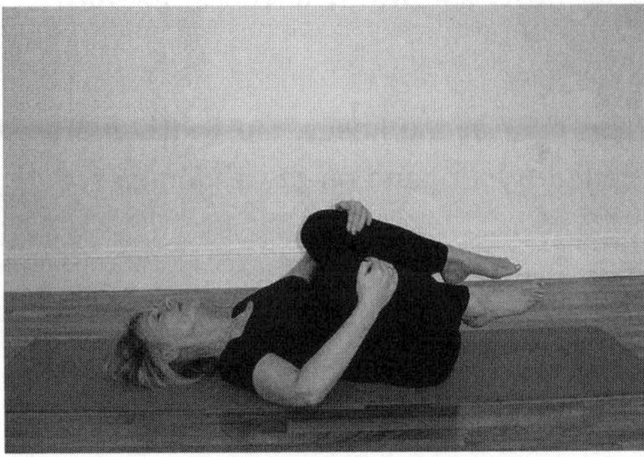

Rocking from side to side

The above exercises are all excellent ways of easing and stretching before you start your full yoga session. In the next chapter we will be looking at yoga postures that are specifically designed to give you more energy and vitality.

postures to **energise** and **revitalise**

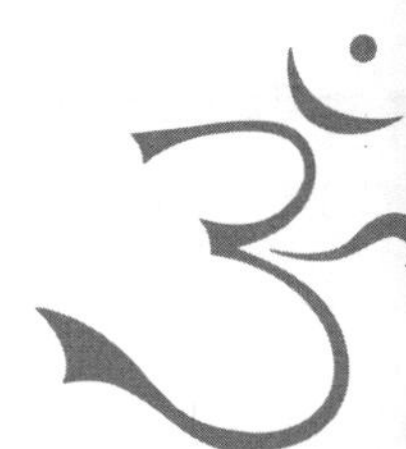

Now that you have relaxed, stretched and warmed up, you are ready to start practising the poses.

Lying Down Postures

Head to Knee Pose *

This is a gentle forward stretch, so you need to counter this movement with a backward bend. This pose helps to tone the bowel and to prevent constipation, wind and irritable bowel syndrome.

1 Lie on your back with your legs out straight.
2 Now bend your right leg and bring it towards your chest, hugging it in by clasping just below the knee joint. Keep everything relaxed on your left side. Squeeze the knee into your abdomen on the out-breath, then release on the in-breath. Repeat five times.

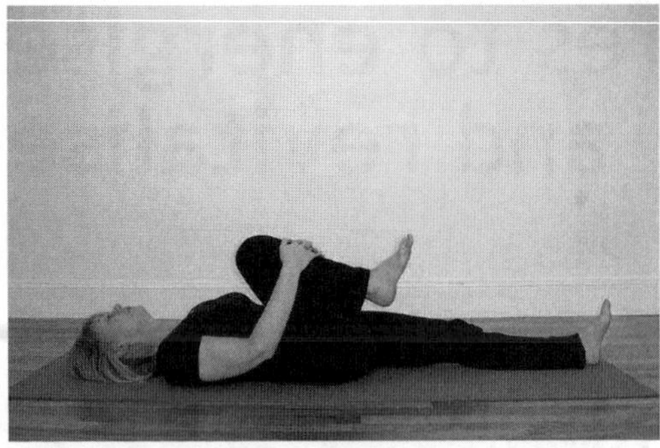

Knee raised, head down

3 Next on an in breath and taking special care if you have neck or shoulder problems, lift your head up towards your knee Hold for a few seconds, breathing normally. Relax your shoulders.

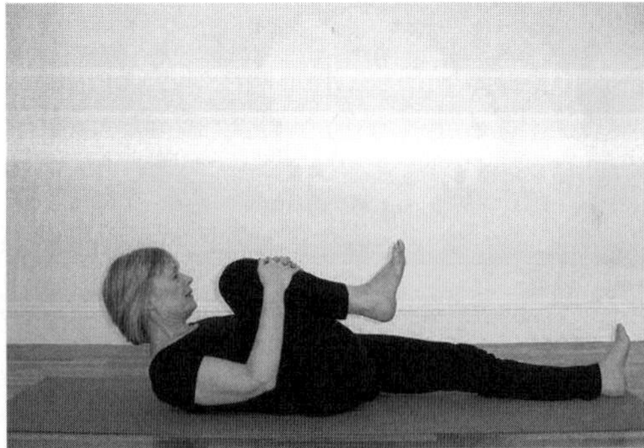

Head lifted

4 On an out-breath, lower your head, then breathe in. On another out-breath, lower your knee and stretch your leg out straight.
5 Repeat three times then do the same on your left side.

Leg Raises

*

1 Lie down on the floor on your back with your legs stretched out.
2 On an in-breath, slowly lift your right leg towards the ceiling. keep your leg as straight as possible and bring it as near as you can towards your head without straining. If you find this too much, you can bend your left leg, which will make the pose easier. If, on the other hand, you are quite supple, you can hold onto your lower leg with your hands and gently bring your leg further towards your head to increase the stretch. Flex your foot towards the ceiling so that your heel is stretching up, which will also increase the stretch. Breathe out. If you are not very flexible use a belt to help you stretch.

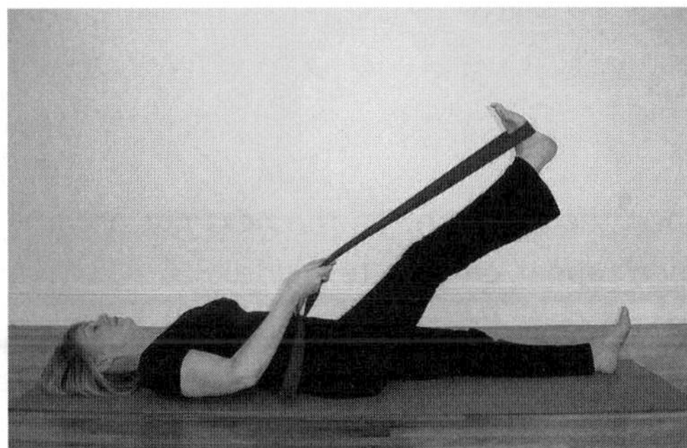

Leg raised

3 Now, breathing in and holding onto your leg, gently lift your head up towards your leg and stretch your leg further towards your head. If you have any neck or shoulder problems do this last part carefully.

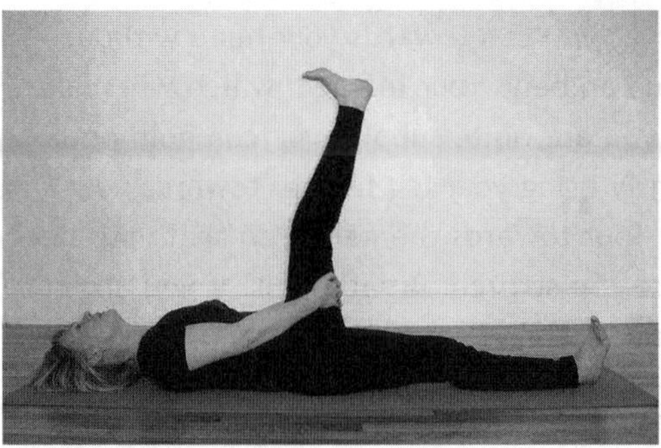

Leg held with hand

4 On an out-breath, lower your head and breathe in. Then, on the next out-breath, slowly lower your leg. Do twice more, then repeat on your left side.

The Fish

The Fish is a backward-bend movement so is therefore a very useful counter posture for forward bends such as the Head to Knee Pose. It is also used as a counterpose to the Shoulder Stand and the Half Shoulder Stand, which I will be explaining later. The Fish is an excellent posture for increasing vital energy to the Heart Chakra because it opens the chest fully. It is also a good posture for breathing problems such as asthma and can help to correct hunched or rounded shoulders.

1 Sit upright with your legs outstretched and lean back on your elbows and forearms so that they are supporting you. Have the tops of your hands under your buttocks.

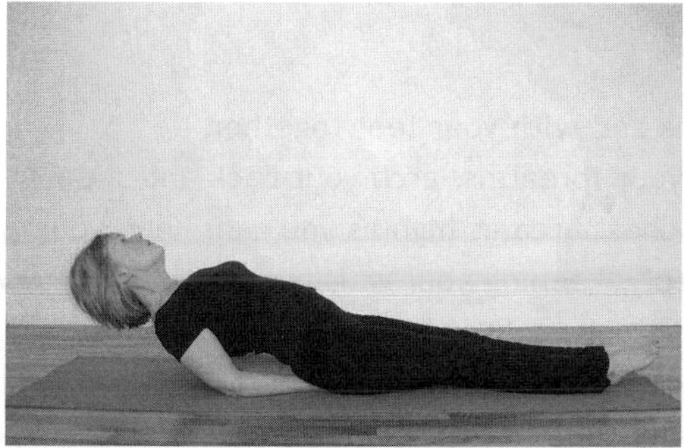

Seated leaning back

2 Pull in the back of your pelvis. Look up at the wall and curve the back of your waist. Look higher up the wall to curve your spine in towards your shoulder blades.

3 Finally, ease your elbows a little further forward towards your hips until you can gently bring the crown of your head to rest lightly on the floor, or on blocks or books. Keep your neck free of any tension. The pressure on your head must be light – your arms should be taking most of your weight.

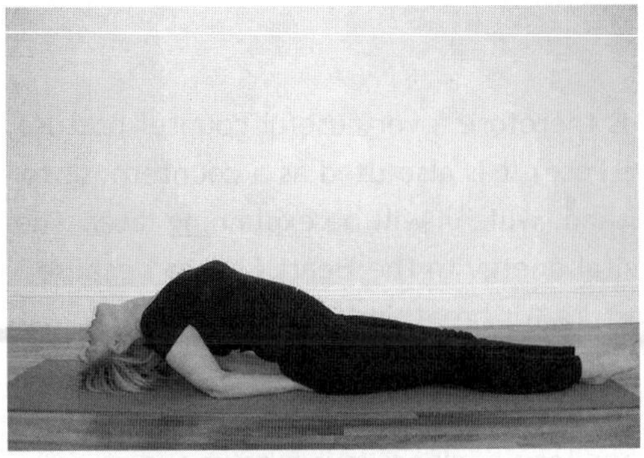

Crown of head touching floor

To work on this posture from the floor when you are more experienced, you can try this:

1 Lie on the floor resting on your forearms and with your feet together.
2 Now, on an in-breath, press slightly on your forearms, arch your back and slide onto the back of your head. Raise your chest area as high as you can. Keep your legs as relaxed as possible. Breathe deeply, keeping your waist area held in.
3 To make the posture stronger push your elbows into the floor to help open the chest even more. Remember, you should not be putting too much pressure on your head. Hold for 30 seconds, increasing this time only when you feel able to do so without straining. Keep your neck relaxed.
4 Breathe out to come out of the posture.

The Bridge

This back bend resembles the span of a bridge. It is excellent for tightening the abdominal area, strengthening the back and keeping the spine flexible.

1 Lie flat with your knees bent and your arms by your side, palms face down. Your feet should be about hip-width apart. Keep the chin into the chest.
2 Keeping your feet on the floor, with your ankles under your knees, breathe in and slowly lift up your hips and move onto your shoulders so that you form an arch. Keep your neck and head on the floor. Tighten behind your knees, thighs, buttocks and lower back. Use your arms to support you by keeping them pushed down under your 'bridge', and press down hard with your feet. Lift your hips as high as you can. If you want to increase the lift, you can hold under your waist with your hands and push up, which will take you further onto your shoulders. Remember to breathe normally and hold the pose for a few seconds.

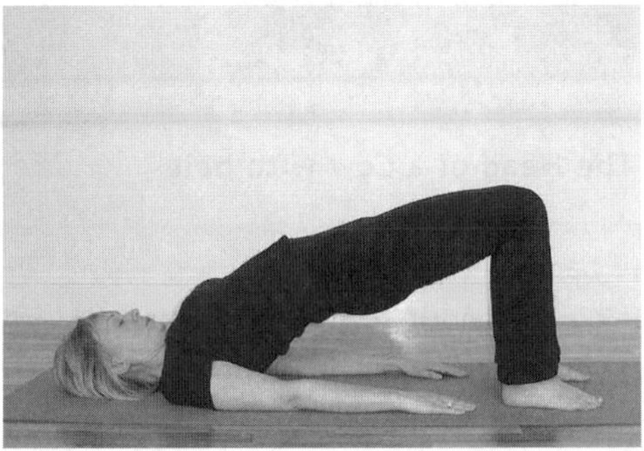

The Bridge

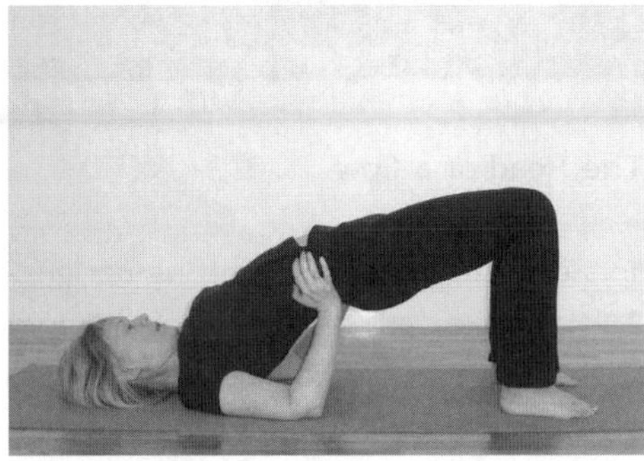

The Bridge - variation using the hands for support

3 Come out of the posture on an out-breath, rolling your back down very slowly, vertebra by vertebra, onto the floor. Repeat twice more. To counterpose hug the knees over the chest.

Sitting Postures

The Head of a Cow

*

Like the Fish, this posture is very good for opening out the chest area and bringing vital energy to the Heart Chakra. It is also good for toning the upper part of the arm. It benefits the shoulders and gives an excellent diagonal stretch to your back.

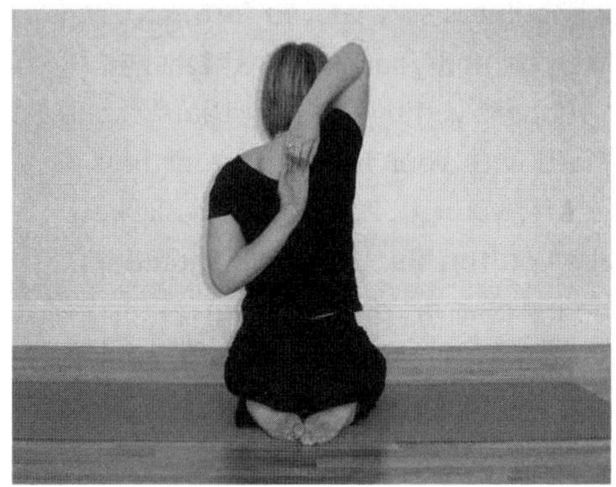

The Head of a Cow

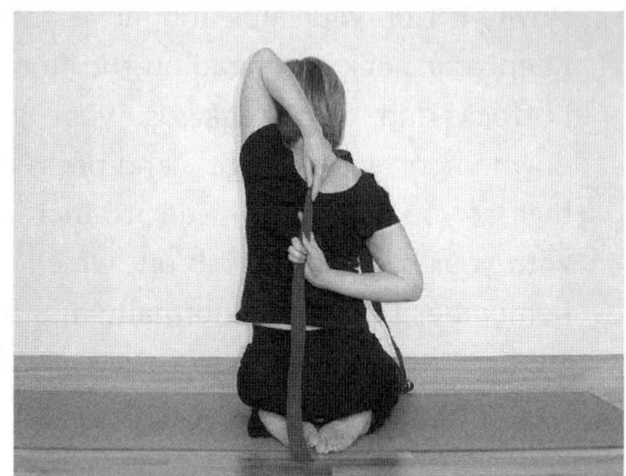

The Head of a Cow with belt

1 Kneel so that you are sitting upright on the back of your heels.
2 Now take your left arm up behind your back and bend it so that your hand is between your shoulder blades, pointing up your back as far as it can reach.
3 Take your right hand down over your right shoulder so that the hands meet and you can grip your fingers together. If you can't reach this far, don't worry – use a belt, handkerchief or sock between your two hands.
4 Pull up and down on your hands to increase the diagonal stretch in your back. Hold for about ten breaths. Now repeat on the other side.

Most people can reach further on one side than the other. This is because it is usually more difficult to twist your dominant arm (i.e. the right if you are right handed) into the upward position.

Sitting Forward Stretch

This is a forward bend, so will need to be counterposed with a backward bend.

1 Sit on the floor with your legs outstretched. Try and sit upright but without any tension in your back – in other words, don't slump. keep your heels together and your toes flexed.
2 Now inhale, raise your arms up over your head and, bending back slightly, look up at your hands. Exhale and slowly bend forward from the hips – not the waist – so that your breastbone is in line with your legs. Just bend a little way and then, on an in-breath, raise your arms up over your head again and stretch up.

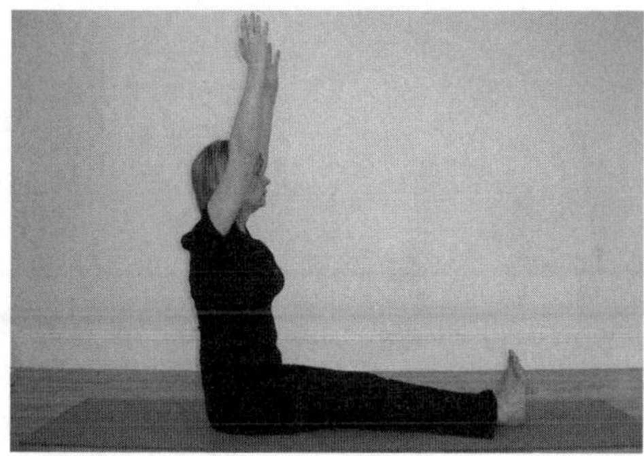

Arms raised up

3 Now, bending from the hips again on an out-breath, fold forward a little further Come up again on an in-breath, stretch your arms up further towards the ceiling then fold your arms and trunk down as far as you can on the next out-breath, keeping your spine in a straight line. If you are very flexible, you will be able to rest your trunk on your thighs and your arms on your calves, or even the floor. Breathe normally and relax.

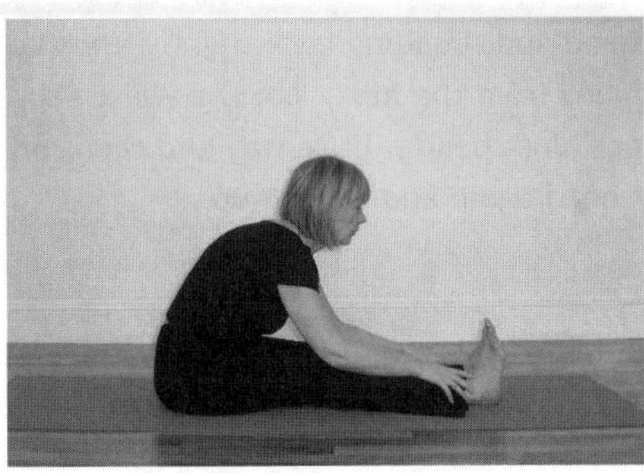

Arms and trunk folded down

4 If you can't stretch this far forward, don't worry – just go as far as you can. You are aiming to keep your trunk straight whilst stretching forward, so don't curve your spine in order to get further.
5 Hold for a few seconds, relaxing and breathing deeply: this helps to generate energy in your Solar Plexus Chakra. Come out of the posture slowly on an in-breath.

This forward bend benefits your internal organs and the nervous system. Whilst performing this posture, remember the saying that applies to all yoga: 'Don't sprain -if pain, no gain!' Listen to your body and work with the principle of 'ahimsa' - meaning non-violence.

The Lion

*

This pose is called the Lion because that is what you'll look like - you make a really fierce face! It is very beneficial if you are suffering from a sore throat or feel you are about to get a cold. It also stimulates blood and vital energy to your face, helping to counteract feelings of lethargy. It will actually help to make you a better colour if you are usually very pale. It's not difficult to do - and is particularly good if you have CFS.

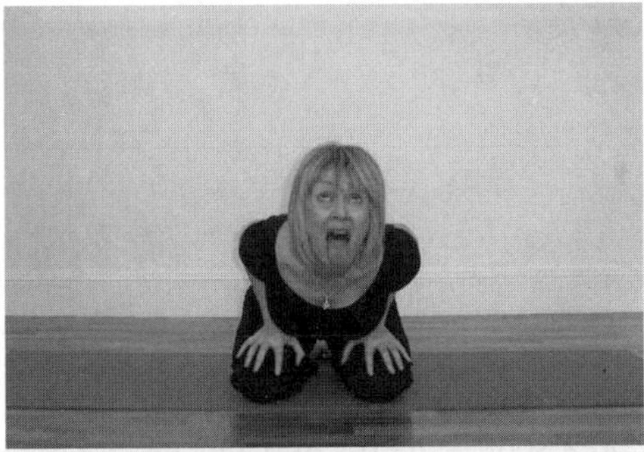

The Lion

1 Kneel resting upright on the backs of your heels Alternatively, sit with your legs crossed. Place the palms of your hands on your knees, with your fingers splayed, and take a deep breath in through your nose.
2 Now lean forward slightly and breathe out forcefully through your mouth, making a 'haaa' sound. As you do so, stretch your tongue out and down, stretch out your fingers, and look up to the point between your eyebrows.
3 Hold the pose for a few seconds then close your mouth and breathe normally. Repeat twice more.

The Boat

**

This posture is very good for firming your abdominal muscles and your back, which in turn will help to support your spine.

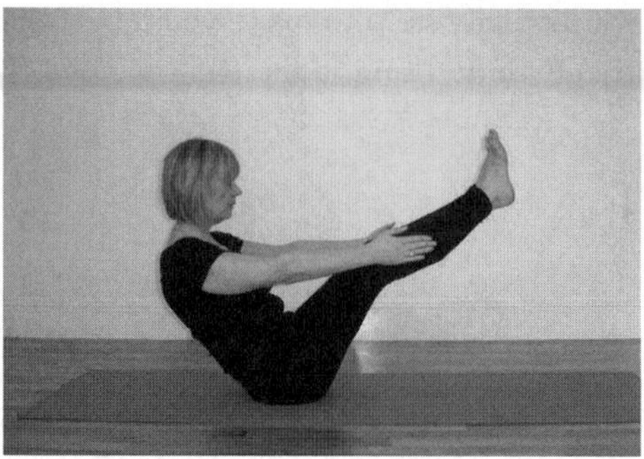

The Boat

1 Sit upright on your sitting bones. Bend your knees and lift the feet off the floor, holding one hand around each sole. Focus on a spot to help you balance.
2 Now breathe out, and on the next in-breath, take your legs up into the air. Your feet should be slightly higher than your eye level. You should be resting on the base of your spine so that your body forms a V-shape. Release your arms so that they stretch out in front of you, outside your legs. Hold the posture for a few seconds – you should feel your abdominal muscles working. Breathe deeply.
3 To increase prana or vitality, make rowing motions with your arms. This helps to pump energy into your body, particularly your Solar Plexus Chakra, which is your energy or sun centre.
4 To come out of the position, reverse the movements on an out-breath. Repeat twice more.

The Butterfly

The Butterfly is a good posture to practise in preparation for the Lotus position. I won't be covering the Lotus position in this book, but if you join a yoga class, you will be taught the Half Lotus and, when you are very advanced, the Full Lotus. (In the Half Lotus, you sit cross-legged with one foot tucked up by the opposite thigh.) Sitting upright helps prana to flow along the spine, and this posture helps ankles, knees and hips to become more flexible.

1 Sit upright on your sitting bones – i.e. not slumping on the base of your spine but sitting up on your buttocks. Clasp your feet together
2 Now, gently bounce your knees up and down. You are aiming to get your knees as near to the floor as you can, and it will help if you visualise your knees going further as you practise this.
3 Do this movement for about two minutes, then put an elbow on each knee and gently press them down.

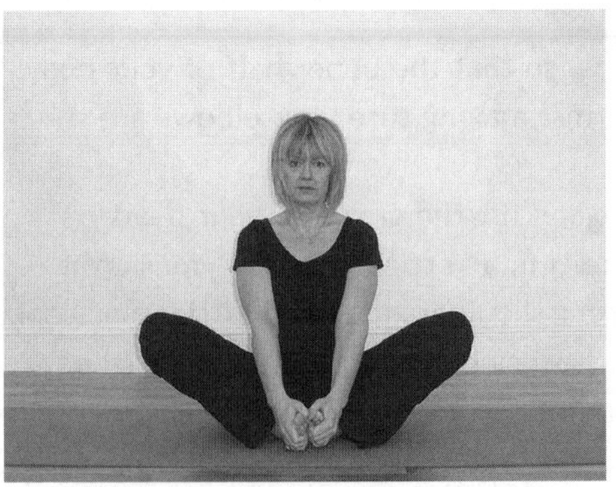

Bouncing the knees gently

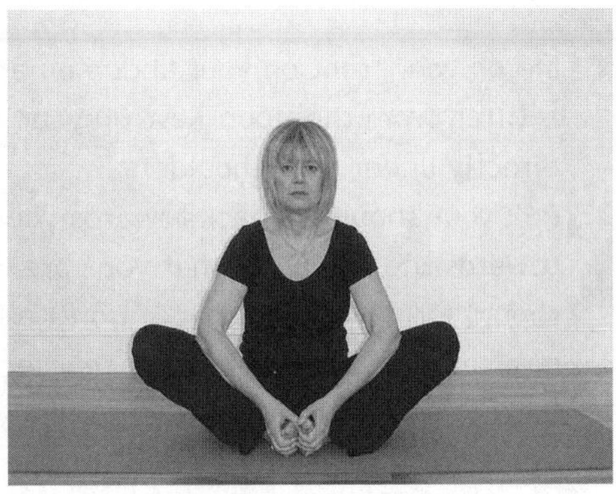

Pressing down gently

Backward Bends

As I mentioned in Chapter 5, backward bends are very energising. They are also used to counter forward-bend movements such as the Sitting Forward Stretch.

The Sphinx *

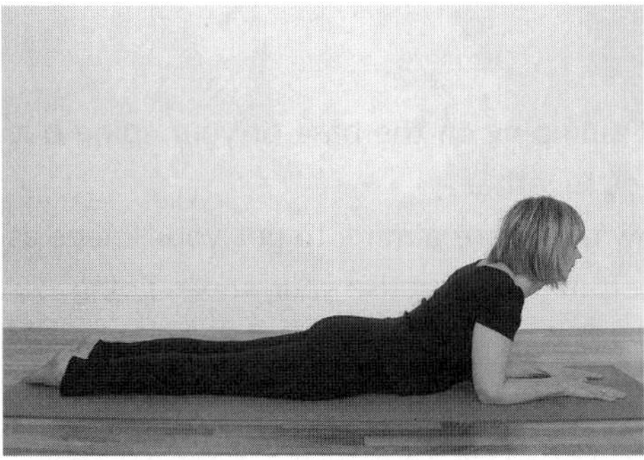

The Sphinx

1 Lie on your front on your abdomen and hips, so that the upper half of your body is lifted from the floor. Rest on your forearms, making sure your elbows are directly under your shoulders.
2 Pull your shoulders back towards your feet and lift the crown of your head towards the ceiling so that your breastbone is in a vertical position. Your arms should form a square shape. Don't allow your shoulders to slump or tighten. Look straight ahead and hold for a few seconds, focusing on your lumbar area (the base of your spine). Breathe normally.
3 Come down slowly on an out-breath, rest, and then repeat twice.

The Cobra **

When you are confident enough with the Sphinx, you can progress to this next posture. This is quite a strong backward bend so it should follow a forward bend, or be followed by one.

The Cobra is very beneficial: it can help to alleviate menstrual problems, to stimulate the adrenal glands and the kidneys, and to improve spinal strength and flexibility – and therefore posture. It generates energy in both the Heart and the Root Chakra. If you have CFS and experience swings of energy or sometimes feel hypermanic, I suggest you stick to the Sphinx and avoid the Cobra.

The Cobra looks simple but it is very easy to get wrong. Don't be tempted to push yourself up with your hands thus compressing the curve at the back of your waist. Your upper back should be lengthened – keep in mind the image of a snake as you practise this.

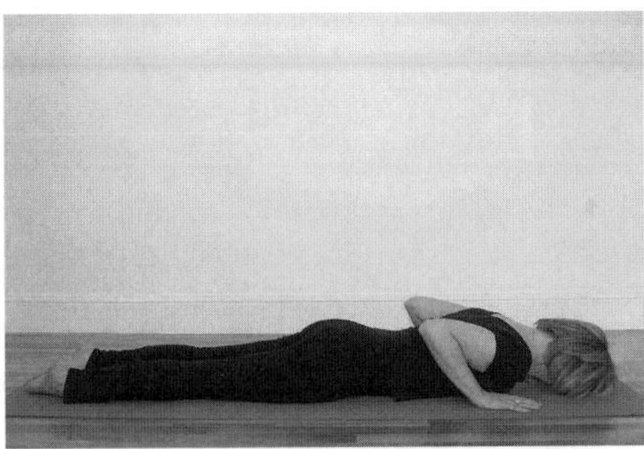

Preparation for the Cobra

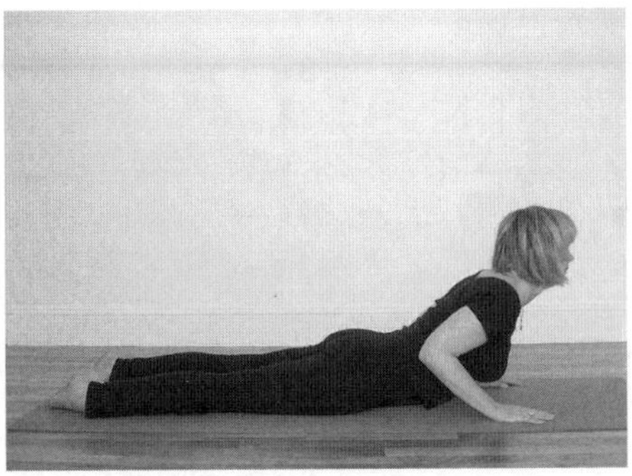

The Cobra

1 Lie down with your forehead on the floor, arms by your side with your palms facing up. Now rest your forearms and palms on the floor under your shoulders. If you haven't done this posture before, put your hands wherever is comfortable, which may be in front of your shoulders. As you progress, you can move your hands nearer your chest, or under your shoulders with your fingers facing forward.

2 On an in-breath, slowly start to lift your trunk. Lift from the hips using your back muscles, rather than pushing up with your hands. As you lift, brush your chin and nose along the floor so that you are leading with your head. Drop your hips and lengthen forward as you lift the upper part of your body, opening your chest and abdomen. Try and keep your shoulders dropped and soft, not hunched or stiff. Look up to the space between your eyebrows and breathe normally. Keep your elbows in.
3 Hold the posture for a few seconds then reverse the procedure slowly to come down. Relax, and then repeat if you wish.

The Locust

The Locust strengthens the abdominal muscles, aids digestion and gastric disorders, strengthens the lower back, helps the bladder and prostate gland, and is also excellent for varicose veins. It is classed as a semi-inverted posture and helps to bring blood to the face.

Half Locust *

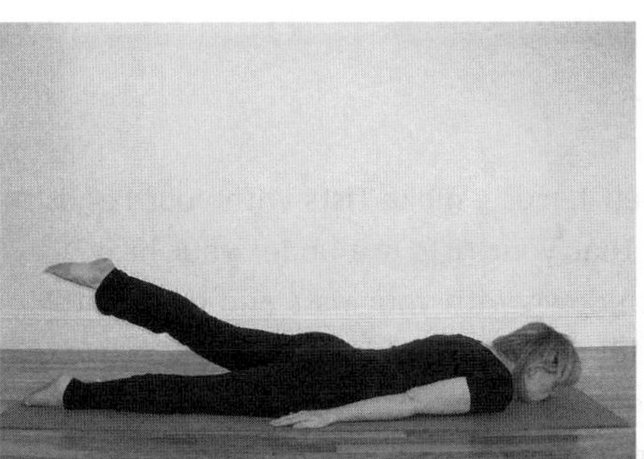

Half Locust

1 Lie on your front with your arms to the side and your palms facing upward. Keep your chin on the floor.
2 Inhale and raise your right leg, keeping the body and leg straight. Exhale and lower your leg. Do the same on your left side. Repeat three times on both sides.
3 Now raise your right leg and keep it up for as long as is comfortable, breathing normally. Exhale and slowly lower the leg.
4 Repeat on the other side, then do twice more on both sides.

Full Locust **

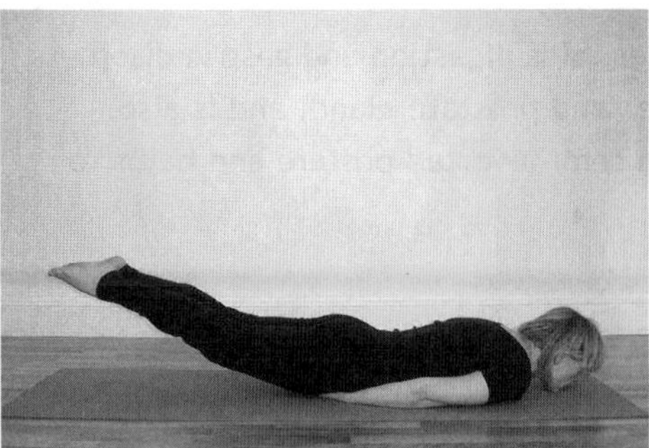

Full Locust

1 From the same starting position as the Half Locust, make fists with your hands and place your arms under your body, so that your fists are under your hips.
2 Keeping your chin touching the floor, push down with your fists and raise both legs from the floor. Breathe normally and hold the position for a few seconds, then on an out-breath slowly lower the legs. Keep the pelvis level as you hold the posture and keep the contact with your hips on your fists.

The Bow ***

This posture raises both halves of the body together, combining the effect of both the Locust and the Cobra. Consequently, it is excellent for toning the back muscles, improving the health of the spine, and increasing energy. It also helps the digestive and reproductive systems and gives the internal organs a massage. It is not suitable if you have CFS, as it is quite strong.

1 Lie on your front with your head down. Bend your knees up so that your feet are towards your buttocks.

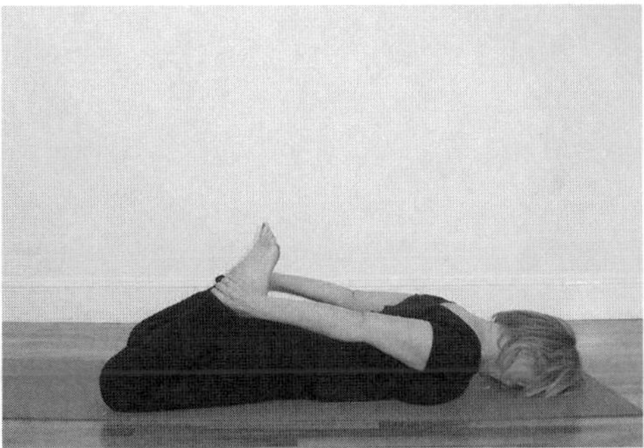

Starting position with feet towards buttocks

2 Now reach back with your hands and clasp your ankles. Breathe out. Inhale and raise your head and chest, holding your ankles. Lift your knees, thighs, hips and lower back so that your knees come up from the floor, your heels move away from your buttocks and your toes point up towards the ceiling. You should be resting on your abdomen. Arch backwards and look up or, if this strains your neck, straight ahead.

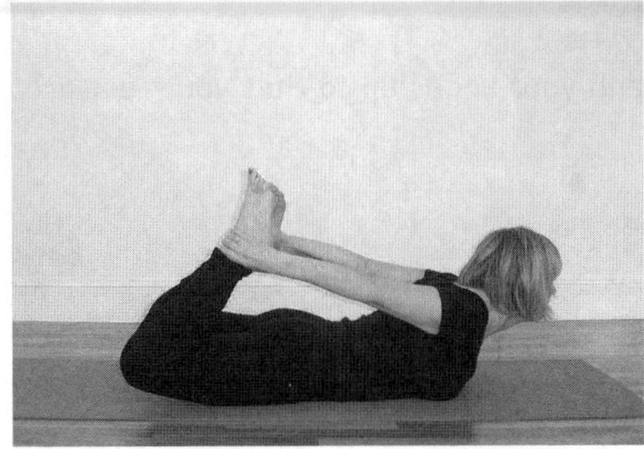

Ankles clasped

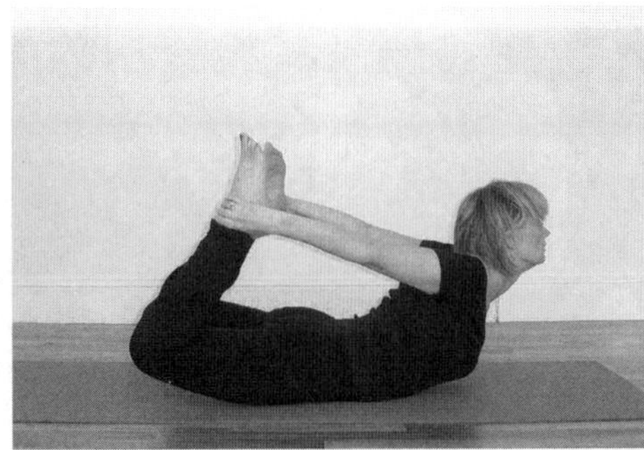

Full pose

3 Take three deep breaths to stimulate energy to your Solar Plexus Chakra; you may find you rock slightly as you breathe in and out. Exhale and come down slowly.

4 Repeat twice more, then relax into the Pose of a Child.

postures to aid **relaxation** and **increase stamina**

7

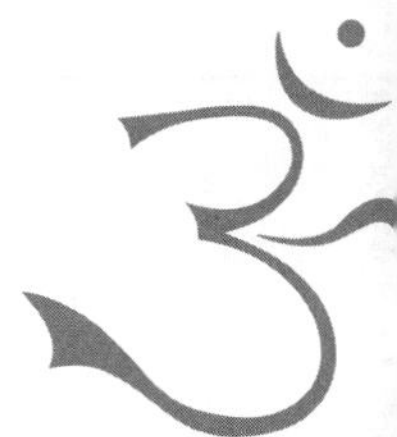

This chapter covers standing postures and twists. Some of these poses are quite strong, so practise them only if you already have a certain amount of stamina and flexibility.

Standing Postures

The Mountain Pose *

This pose will help you to stand with good posture. It is essentially a standing still posture, but don't be deceived – like the Pose of Complete Rest there is a lot more to it, and you need to be completely involved to do it properly. This posture forms the basis for all the other standing postures, and you should try to apply it whenever you are standing during the day waiting in a queue, walking, and so on.

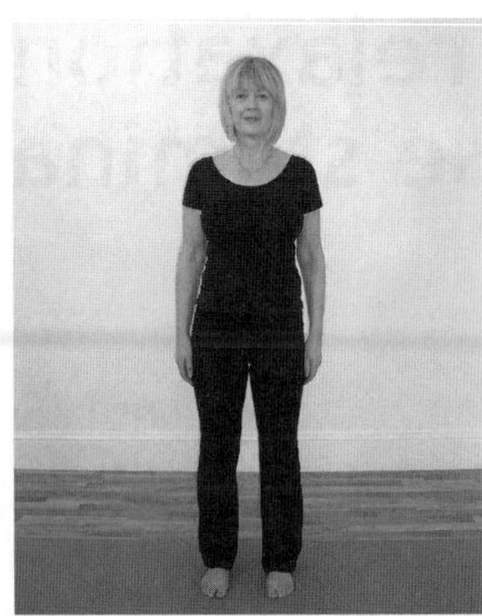

The Mountain Pose

1. Stand up straight with your arms by your sides. Close your eyes. Breathe slowly and relax. Have the feet under your hips.
2. Think about your feet and feel your balance so that you are not too far forward over your toes, or too far back over your heels. Keep your knees soft.
3. Now think about your pelvis. If you wear high heels or carry heavy loads, it is very common for your pelvis to be tilted too far forward. In fact, it should be slightly back, with your bottom tucked under.
4. Now think about your back. Is it straight, or are you rounding your spine? Try and keep it upright without causing strain. Think of your back stretching up. If you were taught that good posture involves holding your shoulders back and thrusting your chest out, this is incorrect for it causes excessive tension. Instead, think about your shoulders being relaxed and falling away from your ears.
5. Now think about your head. Check that there is no tension in your neck and that your head is balanced as it should be – rising up gently from your spine. Your atlas joint, where your head pivots on your neck, is often a point of stress, but because it is a channel for all the main nerves and arteries to the brain, it needs to be relaxed. Your head and your body should be in a straight line, as if a piece of taut string is running up your back and head to the ceiling, with your chin slightly pointing into your chest.

6 Feel yourself rooted in the earth with your feet, with your head lifting up to the sky. You should be aware of how your posture feels, but also relaxed - there should be no tension in any part of you. Breathe normally for a minute or two, then lift your arms up over your head slowly on the in-breath, stretching upwards; then bring them slowly down to your sides on your next out-breath. Repeat five times.

Sideways Bend

*

There are four basic movements of the spine: forward, backward, sideways and twisting. The sideways movement is important because it opens up each side of the chest and abdomen. It is also very good for improving the flexibility of the spine. The Sideways Bend is a very good preparation for the classic yoga pose, the Triangle, which we will be doing next.

1 Stand with your feet apart, toes forward.
2 Inhale, and raise your arms level with your shoulders. Exhale slowly and lower your right arm, sliding it down your leg towards your calf if you can. Keep your pelvis facing forward.

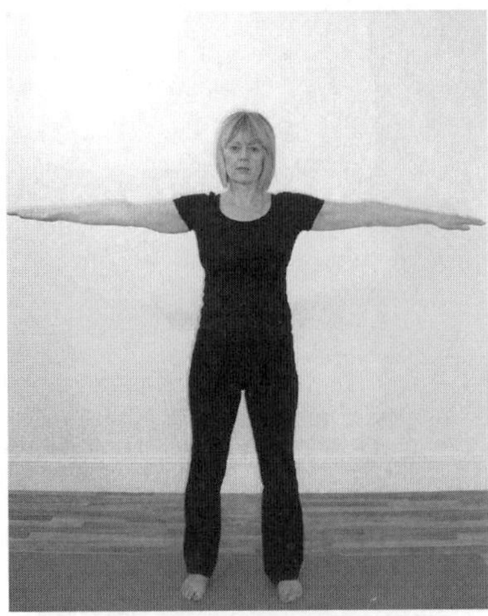

Arms level with shoulders

3 Raise your left arm above your head with the palm inward, so that the arm is near your ear. Bend to the right to take your right arm further down your leg. Hold for a few seconds breathing normally, then inhale to come out of the posture. Repeat on the left side.

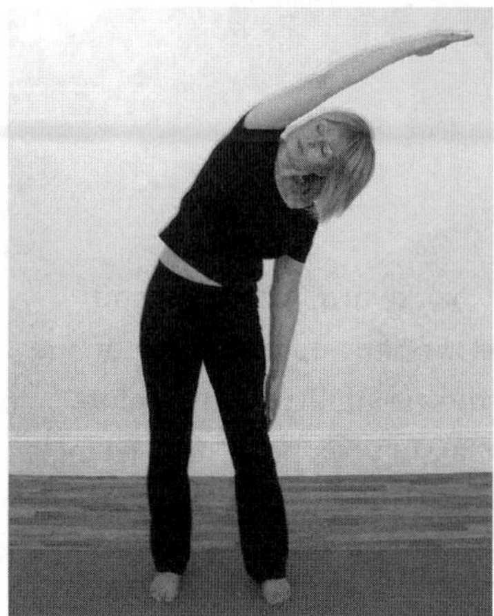

Body bent to the right

The Triangle

*

The Triangle is another pose that looks simple, but is difficult to get right. The temptation is to aim for the floor or your ankle with your hand, allowing the opposite hip and shoulder to tilt forward. If you do this, you won't benefit from the sideways stretch. I would recommend that you practise this keeping your back against a wall, so that you know your hips and shoulders are square-on and facing forwards.

1 Stand with your feet wider than hip-width apart (about 1 metre/3 feet), with your right foot turned out and your left foot turned in just a little. Check that your right heel is in line with the centre of your left foot.
2 Inhale, and then raise your arms parallel to the floor. Turn the palm of your right hand up and push out to the right as if you were trying to push the wall away.

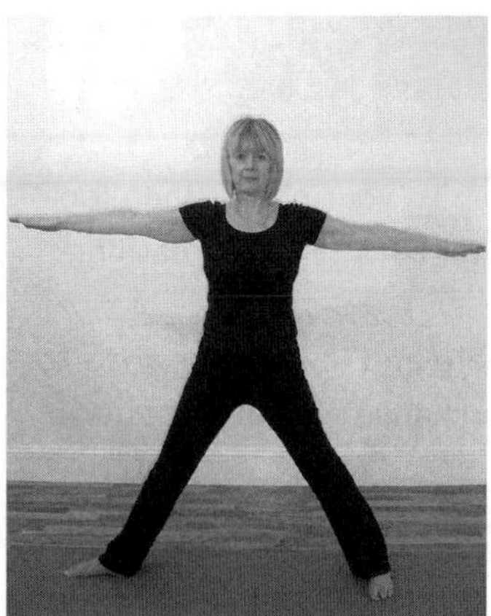

Arms parallel to the floor

3 On your next out-breath, lower your right hand to your thigh and slide it as far down your leg as you can without allowing the left hip or shoulder to swivel forward. Don't worry if you can't get your hand very far down your leg.

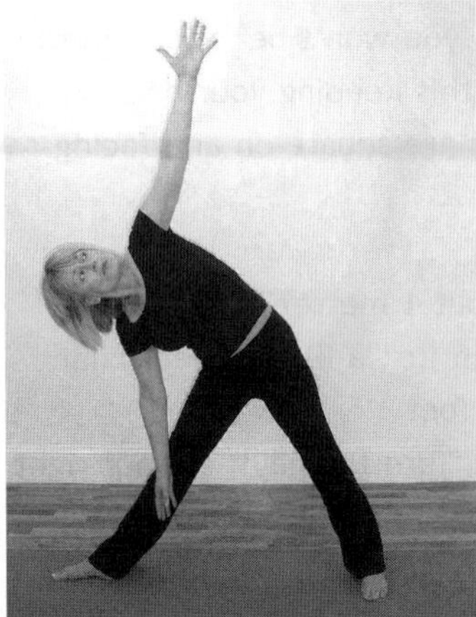

Stretching down

4 Take your left arm up to the ceiling and take your chin to your chest, then look up at your thumb. Remember to keep your left hip well back. Hold, breathing normally for as long as it feels comfortable.

5 Inhale, bring your arms back up to parallel, then exhale and lower your arms to your sides. Repeat on your left side, making sure you change your foot position accordingly.

Standing Forward Stretch

We've already done the Sitting Forward Stretch and now you are going to learn the Forward Stretch from a standing position. This is very useful if you want to counterpose a back bend – and it gives great flexibility to the spine and tones the abdominal muscles. It also helps increase blood flow to the brain, which will give you a huge boost of energy.

1 Stand in the Mountain Pose described at the beginning of this chapter.
2 On an out-breath, lift your arms up over your head, as high as you can.

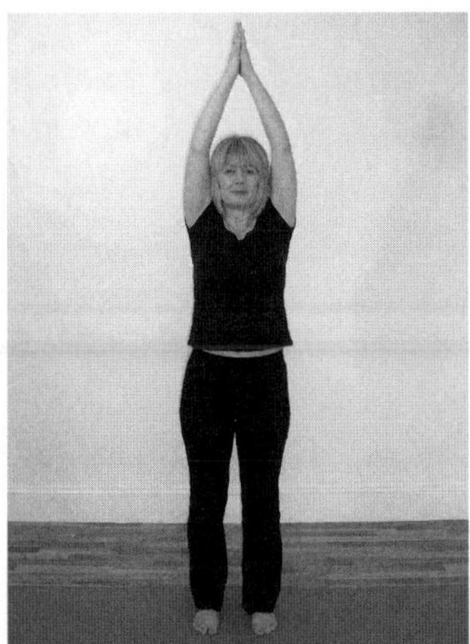

Arms raised

3 On your next out-breath, bend slowly forward from the hips – not the waist – and stretch your arms out in front of you so that they are horizontal with the floor. You can help this movement by pushing your hips and buttocks back to stretch your spine. This will enable you to go further forward and stop you curving your back.

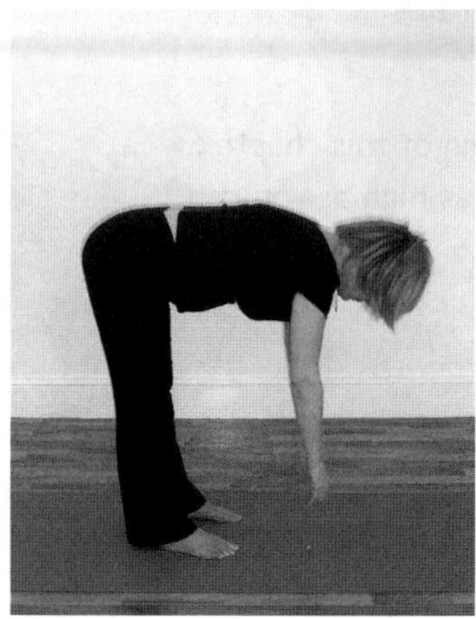

Bending from the hips

4 Now, folding from the hips, come down as far as possible, keeping your back straight. Hold onto your calves with your hands. If you are very flexible, you will be able to reach your feet, or even the floor. Keep your weight forward to keep your legs vertical, and make sure your neck and shoulders are relaxed. Don't bend your knees – reach only as far as you can without straining.

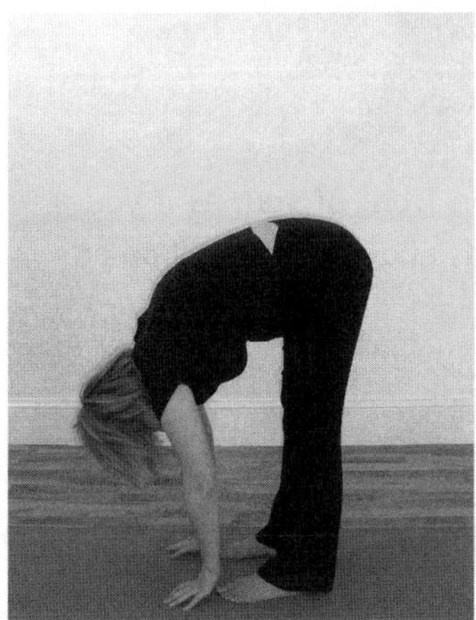

Folding down

5 Hold the pose for about 10 breaths – and each time you breathe out, imagine your head coming nearer to the ground and your chest coming nearer to your legs.

6 On an in-breath, come up by stretching out the arms in front of you and lifting the arms until they are above the head. Uncurl the spine as you do this. Exhale and release.

The Woodchopper

*

This movement is very good for dispelling anger or tension, both of which cause fatigue. It really does work – if something is bothering you or making you really cross, try doing this 10 times and you will be amazed how your negative emotions disperse!

1 Stand in the Mountain Pose with your feet wide apart.

2 Bend forward slightly and clasp your hands together in front of you, as if you were grabbing an imaginary axe. Now raise your hands above your head on an in-breath.

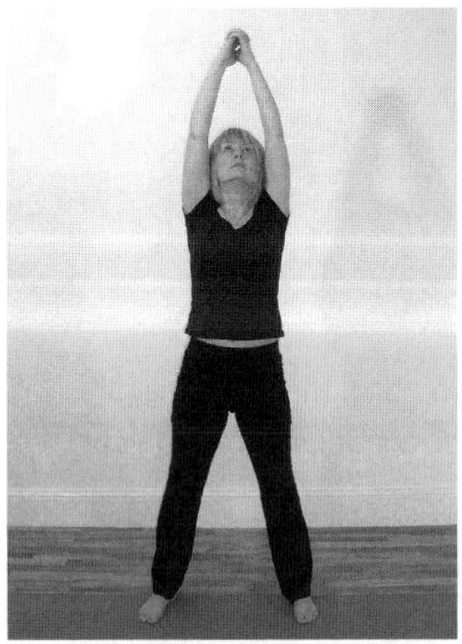

Hands raised

3 On the next out-breath, vigorously swing your axe down towards your feet, taking your arms through your legs and saying 'haaaa' as loudly as you can. Bend the knees as you swing. Repeat five to ten times.

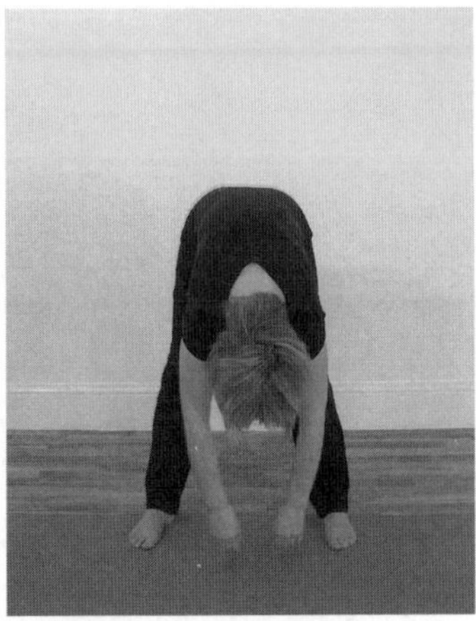

Arms swung down

When you have finished, you may like to relax in the Pendulum pose, which is excellent for releasing tension in the shoulders – another cause of fatigue.

The Pendulum

*

1 Hang forward like a rag doll so that your fingertips are just above the floor

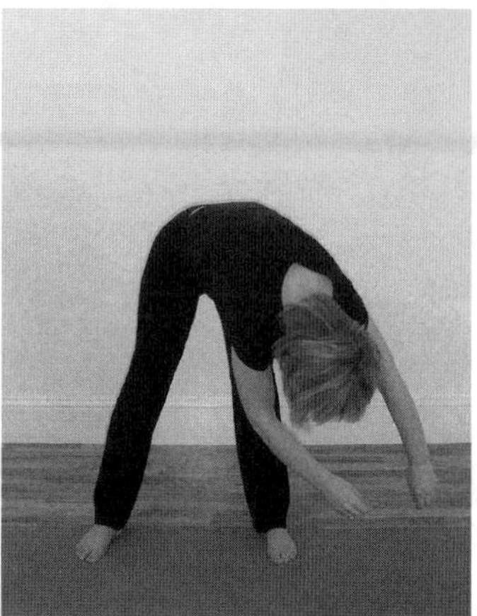

Using your trunk to swing

2 Using your trunk and shoulders, swing your arms from left to right in a rhythmic swinging motion. Then stop swinging and let your arms slow down, making no attempt to control their movement.

3 Wait until they have stopped and then swing them again.

The Tree

*

The Tree posture is very good for balance and for concentration, which is a good discipline to develop before you learn to meditate. It is helpful to visualise that you are a tree, with your feet rooted in the ground and your arms like branches reaching to the sky. This then benefits all your chakras.

1 To get your balance you need to be relaxed and standing in the Mountain Pose. From this starting position you should then be able to stand on one leg without falling over. It will help you to balance if you fix your gaze on something in front of you and concentrate on that point without allowing your attention to wander.

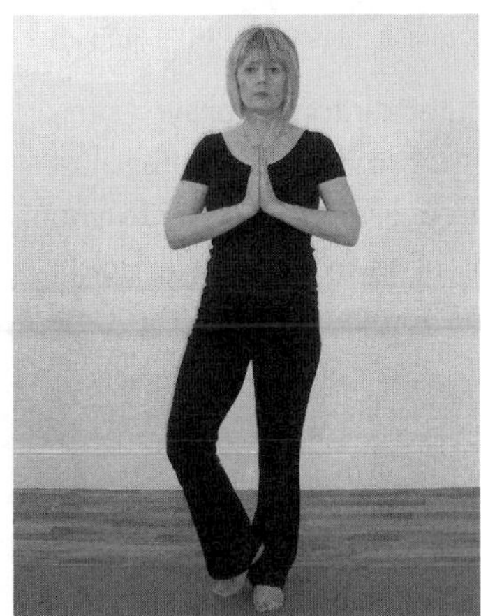

Finding your balance

2 From the Mountain Pose shift your weight slightly onto your left leg. Now take your right leg up and lift the right foot over the left. Find your balance, then lift the foot and tuck it into your left thigh. Tuck your heel into your groin – it's best not to wear socks as the foot tends to slip down. At first, you may need to hold your foot in position with your hand, but try and take your hand away if you can. Try to keep your right knee pointing out to the side and don't allow it to come forward. It may help your balance if you place your left hand on your left hip so that your elbow is out to the side, or if you hold your arms out vertically as if you were walking a tightrope. You can use a wall for support if necessary.

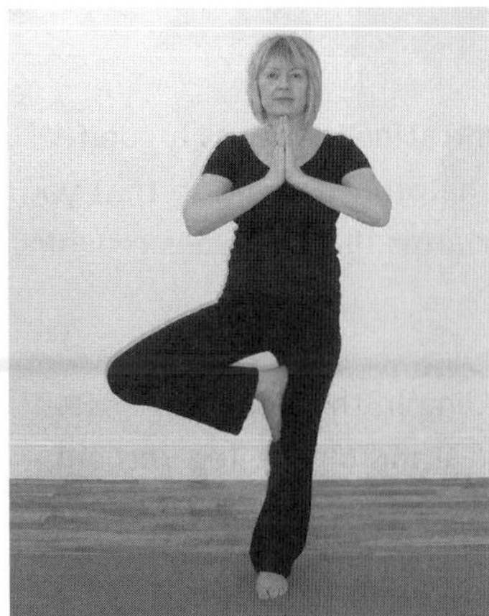

Hands in prayer position

3 When you feel confident, on an in-breath bring your hands into the prayer position and hold them on your chest. Hold for up to 10 breaths, breathing normally, then on another in-breath take your arms up over your head with your fingertips touching. Remember to concentrate on a point in front of you. Hold this position for 10 breaths. As you get more confident you can extend the time you hold your Tree posture.

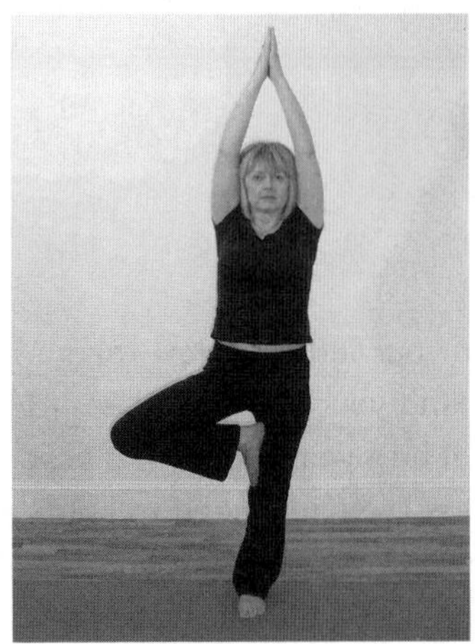

Arms raised up over the head

4 Repeat on the other side.

The Eagle **

The Eagle, a more advanced form of the Tree Posture, twists and squeezes the spine, increasing circulation to the limbs. It will help to strengthen your leg muscles.

1 Stand in the Mountain Pose.
2 Slightly bend your left leg. Now wrap your right leg around your left leg from the front.

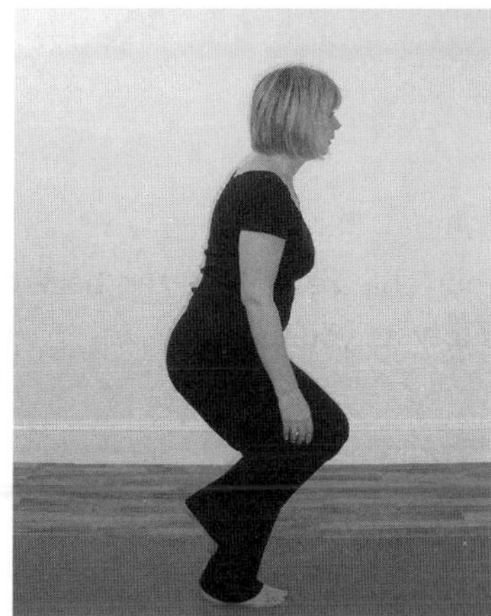

Right leg wrapped around left leg

3 Lean forward slightly and bend your arms so that your palms are facing upwards. Entwine your right arm around the outside of your left arm and hold the palms together. Squeeze your arms and legs together.

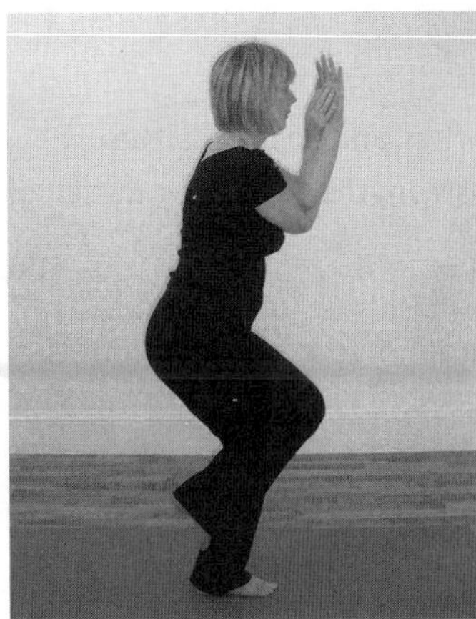

Arms and legs entwined

4 Now if you can rest your elbow on your thigh, with your chin resting on the back of your hand. If you can't do this, just bend down as low as you can.

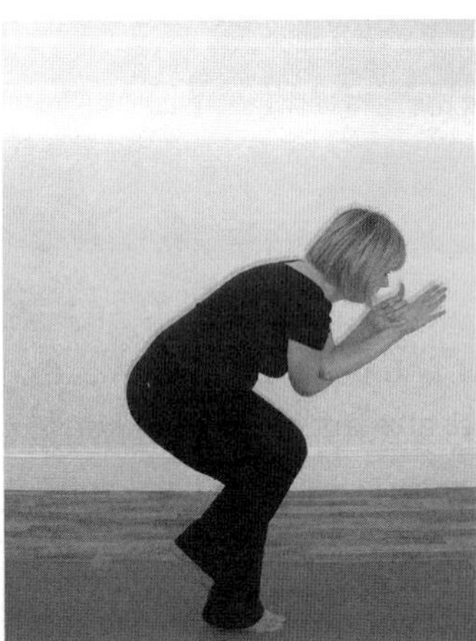

Elbow resting on thigh

5 Hold the pose for a few seconds, remembering to breathe, then untwine. Now repeat on the other side.

The Dancer ***

1 Stand in the Mountain Pose.
2 Take your weight over onto your left leg, spreading your toes. Bend your right knee and lift your foot back towards your buttocks. Extend your right arm back and hold your ankle. Tuck your tailbone under and draw the shoulder blades together.

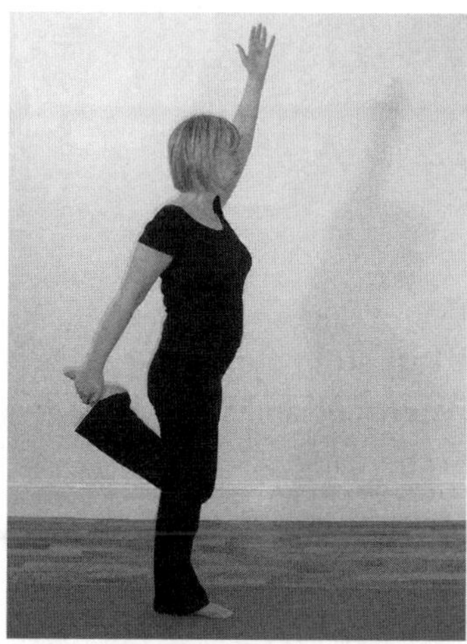

Foot to buttocks and arm raised

3 Breathe in, raising your left arm up to the ceiling close to your left ear, feeling your spine lengthen and keeping both hips level.
4 Breathe out, pivot forward on your hip joints and begin to lean forward slowly, extending the right leg and arm behind and lowering the outstretched left arm to just above shoulder level. Keep looking forward. To increase the stretch, raise your right leg higher on each out-breath. Hold this pose for as long as your balance and breath are steady.

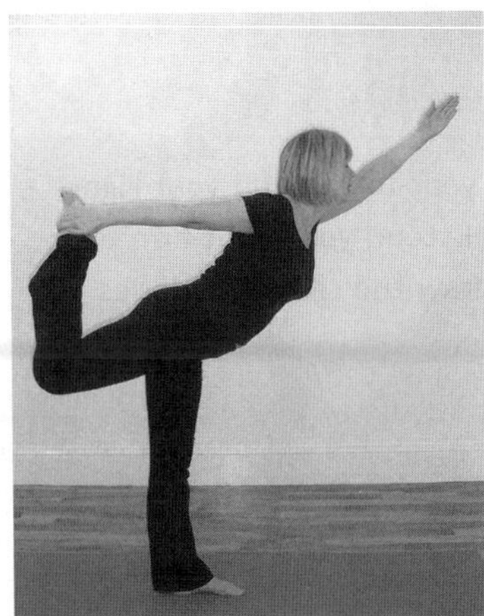

Full pose

5 To come out of the pose inhale then lower your right leg, still holding the ankle. On the next out-breath lower your left arm, release your foot and stand back in the Mountain pose to centre yourself. Repeat on the other side.

Twists

In Chapter 5, I said that for your yoga session you should pick at least one posture from each section. I am including only two basic twists here – a lying and a sitting twist – but it is very important to include a twist in each session as it will both stimulate your spinal nerves and mobilise and increase flexibility in the spine. (You will remember the emphasis I put on spinal mobility and posture and their contribution to your energy levels.) It is also said that twisting the spine stimulates circulation and the internal organs, breaks down fatty tissue, eliminates toxins – and generally increases prana. So there are many reasons to incorporate twists into your daily routine!

The Crocodile Twist

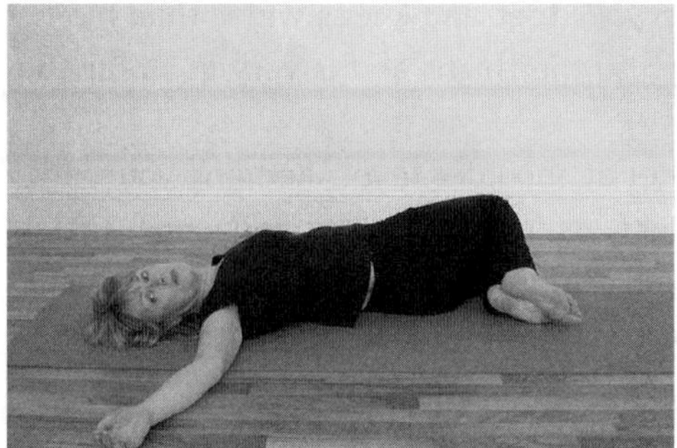

The Crocodile Twist

1 Lie down on your back, with your arms out at shoulder level. Keep your knees together and bend them so that the soles of your feet are under your knees.
2 Now roll over slowly on an out-breath so that your knees are pointing to the right and your left hip is lifted. Look over your left shoulder to your hand.
3 On an in-breath, return your legs and head to the centre, then on the next out-breath, lift your right hip and roll your knees to the left and your head to the right. Breathe in and come back to the centre. Your knees and head should move simultaneously.
4 Keep this a continuous, smooth and slow movement in time with your breathing until you have done about five twists to each side.

Always move slowly and smoothly – don't jerk and always practise on both sides. Remember to breathe out as you turn to the side, and in as you come back to the centre. With all the lying-down twists, it is important to keep your shoulders anchored to the floor while you try to raise your upper hip as far as you can to increase the twist; this gives a diagonal stretch to your back. There are several variations of this movement. You can include just one – or do them all.

Variations on the Crocodile

1 Do the Crocodile Twist as before, but keep your feet and knees wider than hip-width apart. This gives an excellent stretch to the thighs and is very good for the circulation and for eliminating toxins.
2 Lie on your back with your arms out parallel at shoulder level. Keeping your legs straight, cross your left ankle over your right. As in the previous sequence, lift your left hip, twist to the right and turn your head the other way to look at your left hand. Roll back to the centre on an in-breath then twist to the left on the next out-breath, taking your head to the right.
3 Put your right ankle on your left knee. Lift your left hip a little so that your right knee can stretch to the floor on your right side. Turn your head to the left and look at your hand. Now take your right knee over to your left side, allowing the foot to pivot across the knee towards the floor to give it more leverage. Lift the hip and turn your head to look at your right hand. Do this five times on each side.

When you have finished your Crocodile Twists, hug your knees to your chest and rock gently from side to side. As well as being relaxing, this movement massages the lower back too.

The Sitting Twist *

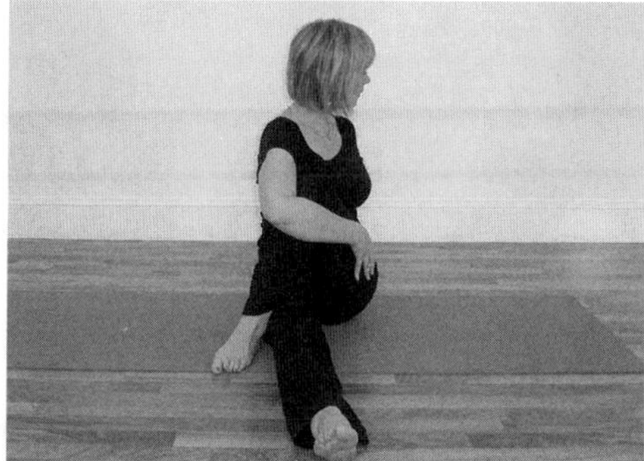

The Sitting Twist

1 Sit on the floor with your legs outstretched. Sit upright on your sitting bones so that you are not slumped.
2 Now bring your right leg over your left leg and place your foot level with the outside of the left knee. Squeeze the right knee into the elbow of the left arm. Raise the right arm to shoulder level, hand and arm parallel to the floor, then sweep the arm around to the right, dropping the fingers behind the spine. Turn your head to look over your right shoulder. Work upwards from the base of your spine so that as you make the movement, your spine lengthens and the right side of your abdomen lifts, followed by your ribs and chest. Sit upright as you rotate your body.
3 Breathe normally as you hold the pose, twisting slightly further round on each out-breath. Repeat on the other side.

In the next chapter we will be learning inverted postures - which are vital for energy - and looking at a sequence that has been designed especially to beat fatigue.

8 postures to beat fatigue

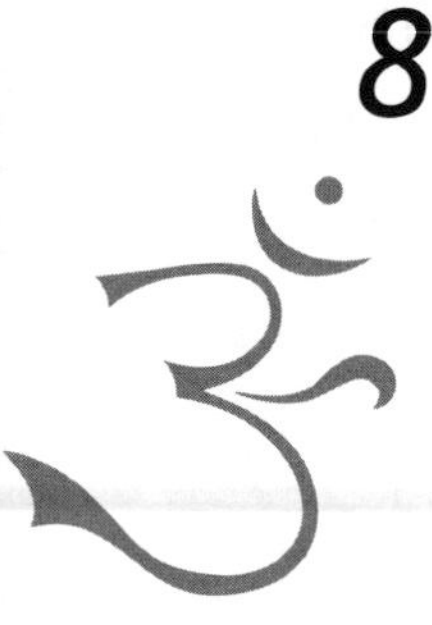

Inverted Postures

In an inverted posture you are either upside down or your head is lower than your heart. These poses are incredibly beneficial in combating fatigue as blood circulation is generally improved and therefore circulation to the brain is encouraged. I haven't included the Headstand because it is difficult for beginners and I think it should be attempted only under supervision, although it is said to be one of the most important of all yoga postures. However, the Full Shoulder Stand and Half Shoulder Stand are just as useful. Both can help remedy a variety of complaints such as low blood pressure, varicose veins and leg aches. They also help to eliminate waste matter in the lower bowel. Best of all, because you have to keep the chin tucked in, the thyroid gland is invigorated, and this in turn stimulates the production of various hormones from the endocrine system, including thyroxine. A lack of thyroxine is linked with poor energy, as you may remember from Chapter 1. Associated with this chin position is a new chakra (identified in the 20th century) at the point between the breast and the neck. It is related to the immune system, which means that the Shoulder Stand can also help to regulate your immune function. The chin position used for this yoga posture also involves the Chin Lock (described in Chapter 4) to help seal in prana and energise your whole system.

All this makes the Shoulder Stand sound too good to be true – a 'cure all' posture – but it really will help to improve your health and energy if you practise it regularly. If you have high blood pressure, or goitre, heart, lung, eye or ear conditions, please check with your doctor before you try any inverted postures. Don't practise these postures if you are menstruating.

Half Shoulder Stand

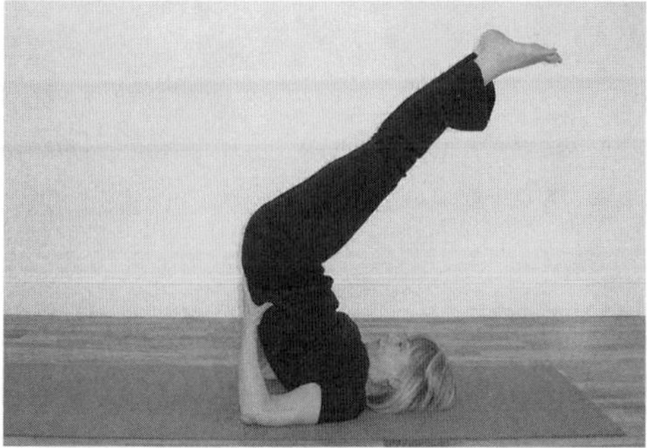

Half Shoulder Stand

1 Lie on your back with your arms by your sides and your palms down. Aim to keep your body as relaxed as possible.
2 Breathing in, take your legs and trunk into the air, bringing your hips off the ground. Immediately support your hips with your hands so that your legs and hips are at an angle of about 45 degrees to your trunk. Work the elbows together as much as possible and move the hands so that they are parallel. Hold this position, keeping your neck and shoulders relaxed, and breathe normally for about a minute, increasing the time as you feel stronger. Keep your legs and toes relaxed. Remember not to strain – if you feel uncomfortable, come out of the posture. If it's easier, rest your legs on a chair. This isn't cheating – you are still getting the same benefits.
3 To come out of the posture, breathe in, and then on an out-breath, lower your legs and slowly roll your spine onto the floor.

Full Shoulder Stand

**

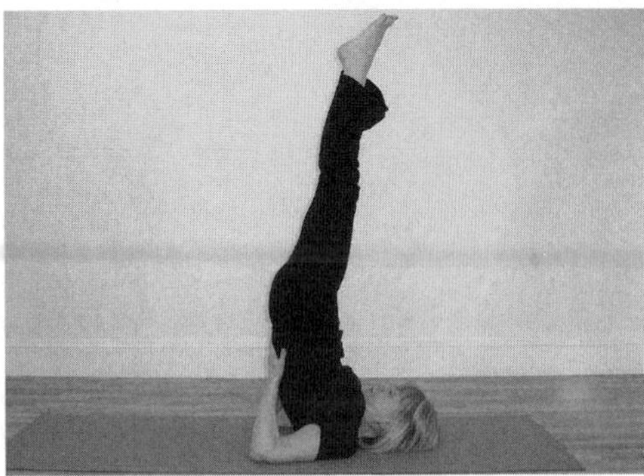

Full Shoulder Stand

Once you have practised and mastered the Half Shoulder Stand, you can move on to the full version of this posture.

1 Lie on your back with your arms to the side and your palms down. Tuck your chin into your chest.
2 Breathing in, swing your legs and hips from the floor. Lift your feet up to the ceiling until your body is straight, working yourself carefully onto your shoulders. Immediately support your back with your hands, keeping them parallel so that your spine doesn't twist. Keep your elbows as close together as possible. Don't sink into your hands but keep your spine as erect as you can, so that you are reaching up towards the ceiling, but without strain. Relax into the posture as much as possible whilst keeping this upright position. Breathe normally.
3 To come out of the posture, breathe out and slowly lower your legs behind you. Arch your neck to keep your head down and roll your spine and hips down slowly onto the floor. Rest for at least as long as you held the posture.

Because you have stretched your neck vertebrae forwards, you must counter this posture by doing the Fish, the Sphinx or the Cobra.

The Pose of Tranquillity

This posture is so called because it can help you with relaxation and is very good for insomnia – try it if you can't sleep at night.

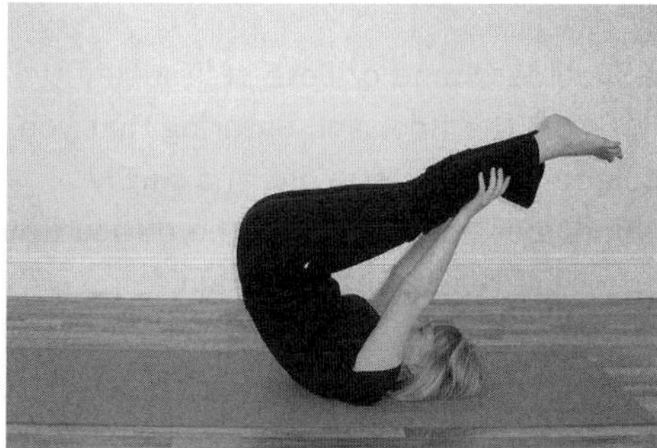

The Pose of Tranquillity

1 Lie on the floor and raise your trunk and legs as described in the Shoulder Stand sequence.
2 Now, on an in-breath, start to lower your legs behind your head – without bending them – until they are at a 45-degree angle to the floor. You should feel a point of balance somewhere between the base of your neck and your shoulder blades.
3 When you feel this balance, bring up your arms and hold your ankles or shins. Hold this position for a minute or two, preferably keeping your eyes closed. Remember to breathe normally. Try and develop a peaceful, floating feeling.

From this pose you can go into the Plough, described next.

The Plough

**

This posture has all the benefits of the Shoulder Stand, but it also gives flexibility to the neck and shoulders, nourishes the spine, releases tension and massages the internal organs.

1 It is best to approach the Plough from the Shoulder Stand or Pose of Tranquillity. From either of these positions, with your hips off the floor and ensuring that you are supporting your back with your hands, keep your legs straight and slowly bring your feet down towards the floor behind your head. This may be difficult at first so just take your legs back as far as they will reach without strain.

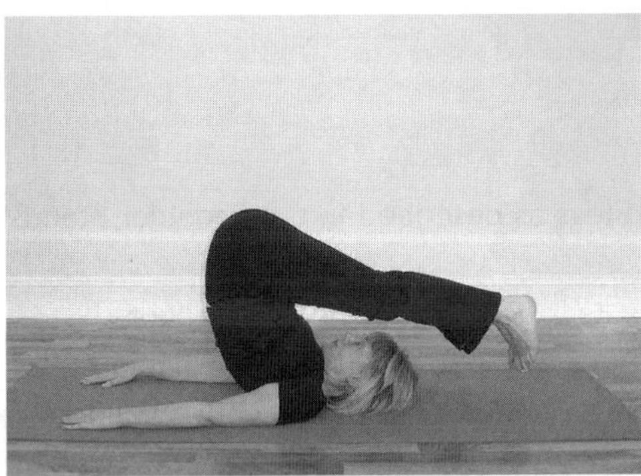

The Plough - preparation

2 When you first learn this posture it is best to place a pile of books or blocks behind your head for your feet to rest on. As you get more flexible, you can reduce the pile and work further towards the floor by pushing your hips back with your hands so that you are balanced on your shoulders. You can then take your hands away from your back and lie your arms out vertically on the floor in the opposite direction to your legs. Try and keep your knees straight so that your legs are parallel to the ground, and increase the stretch by tucking your toes under and pushing back with your heels. Lift your knees.

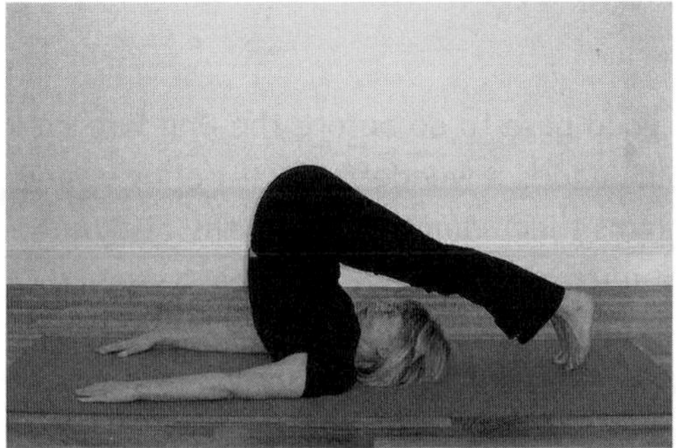

The Plough – completed posture

3 Hold for as long as is comfortable then come out very slowly on an in-breath, rolling down as you did in the Shoulder Stand.

The Cat

*

The Cat is not an inverted posture, but is a good pose to do before the Dog Stretch - which is. The Cat pose mimics a cat stretching and is a wonderful posture for easing the spine. It can help all kinds of back problems – including tension in the neck and shoulders – and generally aids spine flexibility, thereby helping to increase energy.

1 Kneel in an all-fours position with your hands directly underneath your shoulders and your thighs vertical and slightly apart. Keep your back relaxed but flat. Your neck should be relaxed, with your head parallel to the floor.
2 Now inhale, look up and hollow your spine slightly, so that your abdomen is stretching down towards the floor. Press down on your hands. Remember to do this slowly. Hold for a few seconds.

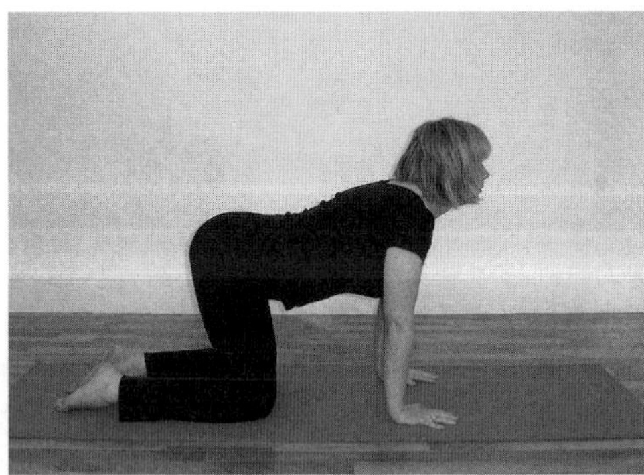

Abdomen stretched downwards gently towards the floor

3 Now exhale and slowly arch your spine up towards the ceiling, as high as it will go. Bring your chin in to your chest Again hold for a few seconds. Tighten your abdominal muscles in the Abdominal Lock.

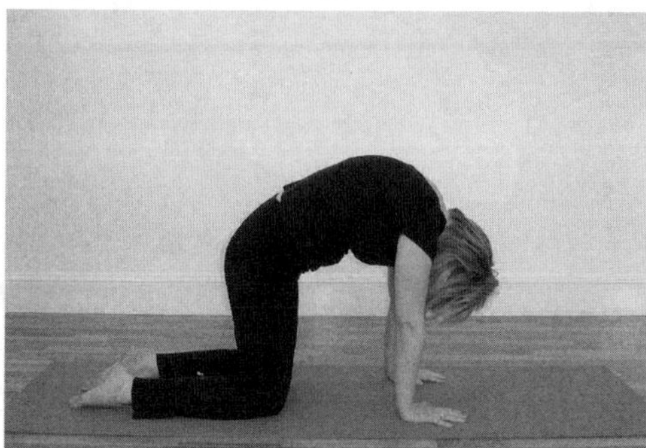

Spine arched towards the ceiling

4 Repeat this sequence 10 times, breathing in slowly to hollow, then out to arch, and timing this movement of arching and hollowing your spine with your breath. Keep your elbows straight throughout the movement.

If you have been sitting at a desk for a long time, or working at a computer, this is a very good sequence to refresh yourself and stretch the spine. Practise it whenever you can take a five-minute break.

The Lying Dog Stretch

*

This is a lovely relaxation posture to use when you have finished the Cat Stretch.

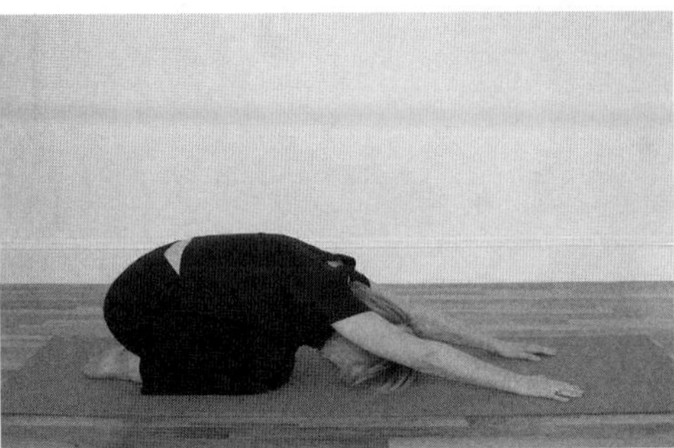

The Lying Dog Stretch

1 From your all-fours position, sit up straight so that your hips are on your heels, then stretch the front part of your body forward, resting your forehead on the floor. Stretch your arms out in front of you.
2 Now relax for a few minutes.

The Standing Dog Stretch *

This pose is great for stiffness and is an effective way to stretch the spinal column, open and release the shoulders, and stretch the hamstring muscles in the back of the legs. You may well have short hamstrings if you lead a sedentary life, which means you will get tired very quickly if you do any walking. Like the other inverted postures, your head is lower than your heart in this pose, which increases circulation to the brain and therefore energy levels. Like all inverted postures, it is contra-indicated if you have high blood pressure, circulation or heart disease.

1 Start from a 'table' position so that you are kneeling on the ground with your hands beneath your shoulders and your thighs vertical – as you were for the Cat. Now move your hands about 5 inches forward. Spread your fingers.

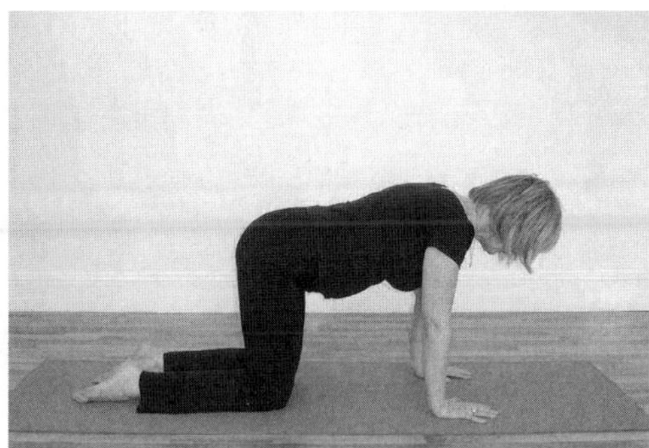

Standing Dog - 'table' position

2 Tuck your toes under and, on an out-breath, straighten your knees and lift your hips up towards the ceiling. You should now be in an inverted V-shape. Exaggerate this movement so that your tailbone is lifting and pointing up to the ceiling to increase the stretch in your legs. Push with your palms, breathe evenly and relax your neck and shoulders. Look at your abdomen. Raise your heels. If you want to increase the lift further, slowly work your heels to the ground, as if you were pedalling. To increase the stretch even more you can ease your abdomen towards your thighs, remembering to keep your hips lifted – don't sink down.

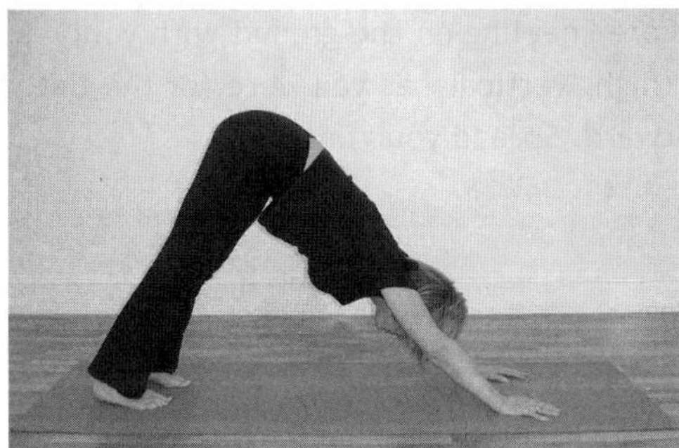

Standing Dog – completed position

3 Hold for as long as you feel comfortable, then come down on an out-breath into the Pose of a Child.

The Rabbit *

The Rabbit, also known as the Hare, has many of the advantages of the other inverted postures but is much easier and quite gentle – so you may prefer to do this instead. It is the first step towards the Headstand and gets you used to holding your head upside down

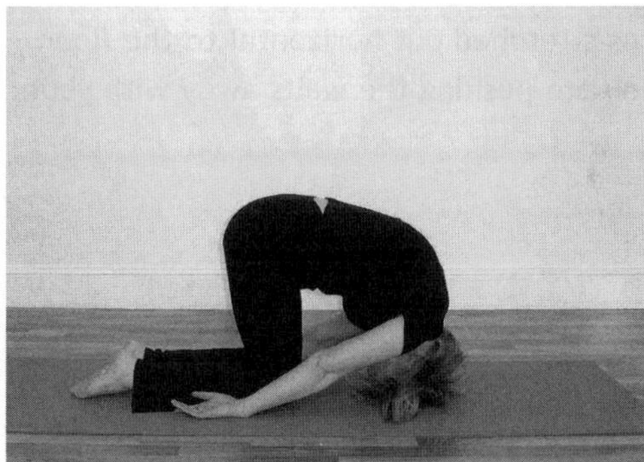

The Rabbit

1 From the Pose of a Child, lift your hips up from your heels and roll onto the top of your head. You may like to put a cushion under your head for this. Hold your shins with your hands or, if you prefer, keep your hands on the floor under your shoulders.
2 Hold this position for as long as you feel comfortable, breathing normally. Rest in the Pose of a Child again for a few minutes, then repeat.

A Simple Sequence to Increase Energy

A yoga teacher, Margo Dixon, introduced me to this sequence. It is a lovely set of postures for making you feel revitalised. If you are doing this sequence at home, you can say the words silently to yourself, but articulating these positive words out loud can have a beneficial effect and help to raise your vitality.

1 Stand in the Mountain Pose with your arms stretched out horizontal to the floor. Increase the stretch by visualising that you are pushing the walls away with your hands. Say out loud: 'I am healthy'.

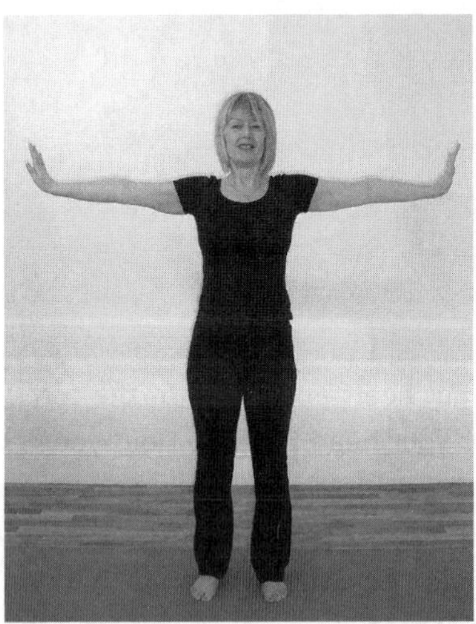

I am healthy

2 Now bend your knees slightly and bend your arms at the elbows with your hands pointing upwards. Say out loud: ‘I am strong’.

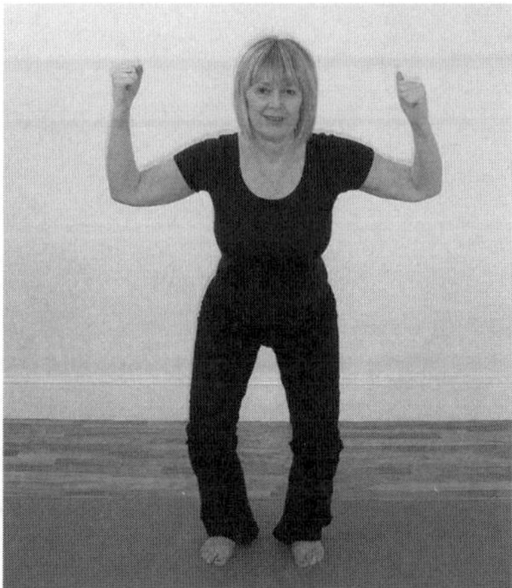

I am strong

3 Next, stretch your arms up to the ceiling and come up onto your toes, so that you are reaching up as high as you can. Now say: ‘I am full of vitality’.

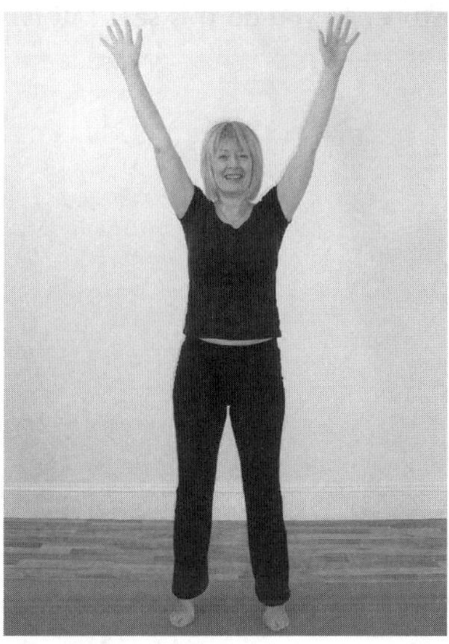

I am full of vitality

4 Come down from your toes and wrap your arms around yourself in a hug. Say: 'I am safe'.

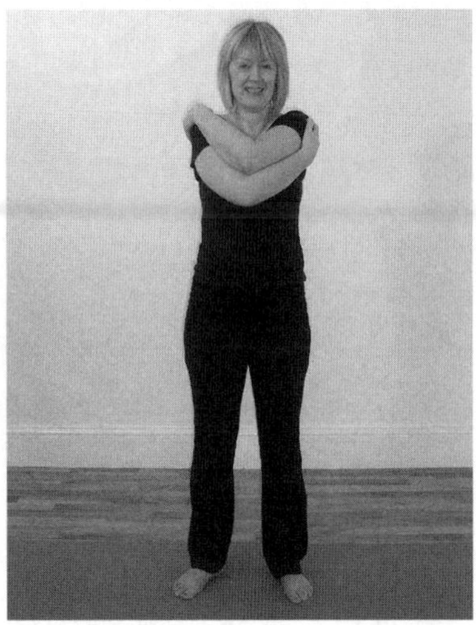

I am safe

5 Finally, come back to the Mountain Pose, circle your arms up over your head, and down by your sides as you did in the Windmill posture. As you do this say: 'All is well in my world'.

Some Suggestions for Daily Routines

In Chapter 5, I suggested that you might like to make up your own daily routines, based on how much time you have, how supple you are and how much stamina you have. Yoga should be tailored to the individual - in other words, choose a routine that suits you.

I am going to give you three sets of sequences that you might like to use if you don't want to make your own. Try to vary these so that you do a different one each time you practise.

Day 1

The Pose of Complete Rest
Quick Tension Reliever
Head to Knee Pose
Leg Raises
The Cat
Half Shoulder Stand
The Pose of Tranquillity
The Boat
Shoulder and neck exercises
The Head of a Cow
The Sphinx
The Standing Dog Stretch
The Lying Dog Stretch
The Pose of a Child
The Pose of Complete Rest

Day 2

The Pose of Complete Rest
Joint exercises
The Butterfly
Full Shoulder Stand
The Plough
The Fish
Sitting Forward Stretch
The Windmill
Sideways Bend or The Triangle
The Sphinx or The Cobra
The Locust
The Bow
The Sitting Twist
The Pose of Complete Rest

Day 3

The Pose of Complete Rest
The Crocodile Twist
The Bridge
Full Shoulder Stand
The Plough
The Fish
Standing Forward Stretch
The Mountain Pose
The Tree or The Eagle
The Dancer
The Woodchopper
The Cobra
The Standing Dog Stretch
The Lying Dog Stretch
The Rabbit
The Pose of Complete Rest

Remember to practise your yoga postures regularly and to visualise prana filling your body with energy. You also need to practise yoga breathing on a regular basis if you really want to see a difference in your energy levels. In the next two chapters, we will look at Chronic Fatigue Syndrome. If you don't have CFS then you may like to go straight to Chapter 11. This will explain how meditation can increase your stamina, make you calmer and generally improve your health at all levels.

chronic fatigue syndrome

9

If you suffer from fatigue, you have probably wondered at some time if you are suffering from Chronic Fatigue Syndrome (CFS). If you do have Chronic Fatigue Syndrome, yoga is one of the best therapies you can use to help you manage and improve your health. First of all, however, let's take a look at what CFS actually *is* as there has been much confusion in recent years about naming and defining this very serious and disabling condition.

Chronic Fatigue Syndrome is the name doctors use to define any unexplained tiredness or fatigue state that lasts longer than six months and which is not linked to exertion, or alleviated by rest. It is sometimes used as an umbrella term to describe the exhaustion suffered with illnesses such as untreated diabetes, HIV, Gulf War Syndrome, heart and lung disorders, cancer, fibromyalgia, depression, multiple sclerosis, post-polio syndrome or post-viral fatigue. More recently, the term CFS has also been used to describe a very extreme illness, which in the UK is referred to as myalgic encephalomyelitis or encephalopathy (ME). Myalgic encephalopathy means an abnormality of brain function, which also describes the various central nervous system abnormalities and cognitive problems associated with this illness. In the US, the term Chronic Fatigue Immune Dysfunction Syndrome (CFIDS) is used to describe the same illness. In the next two chapters, I am referring to ME or CFIDS, but I will use the term CFS to avoid confusion.

What is CFS?

Symptoms include:

- Extreme fatigue after minor mental or physical tasks. An acute reaction is often experienced even up to 72 hours after simple exertion that would seem normal and easy to healthy people. This is not made better by rest. Sufferers may take days or even weeks to recover.
- Muscle pain.
- Severe headaches.
- Malaise – a feeling of being 'poisoned'.
- Sensitivity to noise and light.
- Feeling too hot or cold – a problem with temperature control.
- Dizziness.
- Cognitive problems such as brain fog – difficulty in concentration, problems with memory and attention span.
- Problems to do with the nervous system, such as panic attacks.
- Disturbed sleep patterns.
- Digestive problems – gut dysbiosis.
- A pattern of relapse and remission – some days being able to do more than at other times.

These are just a few of the more common symptoms, but from this you can see that CFS is much more profound than mere 'tiredness', and most sufferers find it impossible to lead a normal life. This is why many people object to the term CFS, as the illness is clearly much more than just long-term fatigue. In a survey carried out by the UK charity Action for ME in 2001, 89 per cent of the 2,300-plus respondents had, at some time, either been bed-ridden or house-bound by their illness.

So, if you have CFS, you will certainly know about it. Most people with CFS find that any mental or physical exertion can produce severe symptoms. On some days you may feel well – you may even have good weeks. But whatever the case, if you have CFS, you will find it impossible to cope with your previous level of lifestyle. This can be very hard. The majority of those with CFS have to give up full-time work and severely curtail their social activities. For some people, even moving a limb or doing a simple task such as having a bath or cooking a meal may seem like climbing a mountain. CFS is total physical and mental exhaustion – like a battery that has gone completely flat. Worse, you don't just feel very tired: you feel unwell for much of the time. CFS can affect anybody, from children through to the elderly, and both men and women of all social classes and ethnic groups. Various surveys in both the US and the UK show that up to 1 in 350 of the population may be affected by CFS. Some people with CFS make a full recovery in time; the majority stay the same, that is, follow a pattern of remission and relapse. A small minority gradually deteriorate.

CFS and Your Emotions

If you have CFS, you may find that you experience a kind of grief – a sense of loss for your old way of life and who you were before you got ill. You may experience shock, disbelief and, later on, anger. These are all normal emotions under the circumstances. The way to improve and to have some quality of life is to move forward and learn to come to terms with the illness. This is where yoga comes in, as yoga shows you how to accept what can't be changed and make the best of what you have. Because yoga is non-competitive, it teaches you not to 'push' but to listen to your body. When you are no longer using up energy fighting the illness but are able to accept that this is how you are for now and that you have to make the best of your restricted lifestyle, you may find that you start to get better. Your self-esteem will rise as you learn not to judge yourself by what you do, but by who you are. You will also be able to appreciate small things – such as a beautiful flower, a sunny day or just time when you are well enough to see a close friend.

What Causes CFS?

The jury is still out on what CFS is. A few years ago, because nothing tangible could be seen under a microscope, some psychiatrists put forward the view that CFS was a psychological problem of 'learned helplessness' - that is, after an initial bout of illness, patients had 'learned' to be tired all the time. This was also referred to as a 'dysfunctional illness belief'. Unfortunately, this did a lot of damage and patients still suffer with the stigma of being labelled 'malingerers', 'lazy', or having a 'psychological illness that is all in the mind'. One author, Elaine Showalter, even wrote a book called *Hystories* in which she suggests that CFS is a cultural narrative expression of hysteria: a kind of modern social problem maintained by some doctors and support groups.

Luckily, we live in much more enlightened times and there is now hard scientific evidence that CFS has a physical origin. Nevertheless, because CFS is a chronic, disabling illness, some people may suffer with depression as a result of the restrictions and pain the illness places on their lives. Yoga, of course, sees us as 'whole' beings. In other words, mind, body and spirit are all linked, and whatever affects the mind or spirit will affect the body. The exercises given later help to address this 'holistic' approach to managing CFS.

It is generally agreed that CFS may be triggered by one or more of the following:

- A viral infection, such as flu, Epstein Barr or other virus, combined with not taking adequate rest to recover.
- A bacterial infection such as chlamydia, mycoplasma or heliobacter pylon.
- Exposure to environmental toxins such as organophosphates or mercury amalgams.
- An inoculation.
- Shock.
- Prolonged stress, combined with one of the factors above.

In 1998, the UK's Chief Medical Officer, Sir Kenneth Calman, said:

'I recognise Chronic Fatigue Syndrome is a real entity. It is distressing, debilitating, and affects a very large number of people.' This was then confirmed in January 2002 when, after a three year study, the UK's chief medical officer, Sir Liam Donaldson, published a report recognising ME/CFS as a 'real' and 'disabling' illness.

The World Health Organisation classifies CFS as a disease of the central nervous system. Current research indicates that CFS is initially a problem of the immune system and that for some reason – perhaps, for example, because of a virus, combined with being run-down and under stress – parts of the immune system do not switch themselves back off again. In this way, the immune system is chronically activated – even if the initial virus has disappeared. There is some evidence of raised levels of cytokines and activated T lymphocytes (parts of the immune function) in some people. This episodic immune dysfunction is, in itself, very tiring. If this scenario continues, it eventually causes damage to the hypothalamic-pituitary-adrenal axis (HPA), part of your central nervous system (CNS). This affects nearly every function in the body. Your CNS is centred in your brain and spinal cord and is made up of millions of nerve cells, or neurons, which send messages around the body. The CNS controls bodily functions such as breathing, heartbeat and digestion, and all sensory perception such as pain, pleasure and the control of muscle movements. An example of this would be how the CNS affects our stress mechanism, or 'fight and flight' response, which we saw in Chapter 1. The autonomic part of your nervous system is needed to switch your stress response 'on' and 'off'. If it is not working properly, this may not happen.

Other symptoms such as fatigue, sleep disorders and poor temperature control are all consistent with hypothalamic dysfunction. The hypothalamus is in the brain, and you may remember that some of the yoga exercises, such as Alternate Nostril Breathing, can help to regulate its function.

Dr Andy Wright, who runs a CFS clinic and is an expert in chronobiology (the science of keeping in tune with our body's natural rhythms) says: 'Heart rate variability studies have shown that there is an excess of sympathetic over parasympathetic tone. This means that a constant biological stress message is present in the body.' Dr Wright is referring to research which shows that parts of the CNS are over-activated, which, in turn, causes those with CFS to become hyper-aroused to stimulation, which exhausts them very quickly.

I once had my central nervous system tested on a machine called a 'Heart Rate Variable' monitor. The results showed that my CNS was, indeed, dysfunctional. Dr Ian Hyams, who also runs a CFS clinic, asked me to come back a week later to see if I could vary the reading, using yoga techniques. He was amazed when, after a period of deep meditation and relaxation, I showed a much more normal reading. In other words, yoga can help to calm and normalise your central nervous system, which, in turn, is going to have a profound and positive effect on your health.

Dr Derek Pheby, an epidemiologist and member of the UK Government's key Group of CFS/ME, says: 'Such changes have been demonstrated affecting, for example, the autonomic nervous system. Another significant change is in the hypothalamic-pituitary axis, the mechanism by which the brain controls the functioning of the pituitary gland and hence the endocrine system.' This then brings us to your hormone system. Your pituitary gland (part of the HPA axis) is often referred to as the master gland, as it controls all your endocrine functions, and this involves everything to do with your hormone production.

Your hormones are chemical messages, which travel via your bloodstream. They bring together all kinds of bodily mechanisms including your emotional responses. Various trials in America have shown, for example, that many of those with CFS put out either too high or too low levels of DHEA and cortisol, which are hormones produced by the adrenal glands. Research has shown that this constant biological stress causes adrenal fatigue. MR scans of the adrenal glands of those with CFS have shown that there is actually a reduction in adrenal gland size in some cases. You may remember from Chapter 1 the role that your adrenal glands play in dealing with stress. This explains why those with CFS can't deal with pressure very well without becoming ill.

In another example of endocrine dysfunction, some people with CFS may suffer with an underactive thyroid. Your thyroid produces hormones that convert your food into energy and help to convert oxygen into your cells. Your thyroid gland also affects your metabolism, fertility and body temperature. Other hormones, such as melatonin, which affects your body clock and sleep, may also be affected by endocrine dysfunction.

Yoga can help to normalise your hormone system, and many of the postures work to balance the various endocrine glands throughout the body. For example, the Shoulder Stand helps to stimulate the thyroid gland, and some of the backward bends can help to normalise your adrenal system.

CFS, Poor Circulation and Oxidative Stress

Yet more research using brain scans shows that CFS patients have a lack of blood-flow to the brain stem. This seriously affects brain function. Often, someone with CFS who is tired, or has overdone things, will become very pale and find it difficult to concentrate or find the right words. This indicates a lack of circulation to the brain. Blood is literally draining away from the head. All the inverted postures in this book will help to remedy this. This is a reason why I recommend that anyone with CFS does an inverted posture such as the Half Shoulder Stand every day. Generally, yoga will help with mental focus and problems such as 'brain fog' - one of the more distressing symptoms of CFS.

Some studies have shown that those with CFS have a reduced capacity to convert oxygen efficiently, which is a measure of aerobic fitness, or how well the body uses oxygen. Again, the yoga breathing exercises given in Chapter 4 will greatly improve your energy, by helping you to convert oxygen more effectively into your cells.

Finally, many experts believe that CFS is related to something called 'oxidative stress'. Professor Majid Ali, a leading researcher in New York, puts forward the thesis that all of the co-factors described in this illness (immune dysfunction, CNS and endocrine abnormalities etc.) contribute to a total burden of oxidative stress. Put simply, the implications of this are that you have too many free radicals in your body, which are then not eliminated properly, because those with CFS seem to have problems with detoxification. This, in turn, means poor oxygen transportation to your cells, poor oxidation in cells, the build up of acids in the body and blocked lymph glands. Your lymphatic system detoxifies your body by carrying waste products out of your system. However, it only moves with your circulation or with exercise. Dr Andy Wright explains: 'Further clogging of the lymphatic system, I feel, could be due to immune hyperactivity.' All the yoga postures work on stimulating the lymphatic system gently, which is why yoga is so effective in detoxifying your system.

To summarise then, if CFS is a disease of the immune system, central nervous system and endocrine functions which contribute to oxidative stress, you can perhaps see why yoga can have such a beneficial effect for those with ME or CFIDS.

To Exercise or Not?

Quite simply, if you have CFS and you attempt too high a level of activity, you will relapse. This can then make you avoid activity altogether, which will bring its own set of problems, such as muscle wastage - and yet more fatigue, because your body needs some activity to convert your food into energy. The subject of exercise is very controversial for those who have CFS. In most cases, prolonged aerobic exertion will push you into a relapse ('aerobic' means an activity that raises your heart rate). In a paper demonstrating the organic basis for CFS, Dr Andy Wright says: 'Giving general advice to simply increase aerobic exercises incrementally often makes people worse. Exercise capacity is reduced. This is partly secondary to an inability to achieve maximal predicted heart rate. This is thought to be due to autonomic dysfunction.'

Dr Cheney, who is Professor of Medicine and Chair of the Nutrition Department at Capitol University, Washington, and one of the leading experts of CFS in America, explains that the aerobic system in CFS is injured and that aerobic exercise past a certain point can dramatically worsen CFS. In the UK, many of the hospitals that treated those with CFS in the 1990s used programmes called 'graded' exercises, where patients were forced to do a bit more physical exercise every day, no matter how ill they felt. This was based on the idea that people with CFS had 'unhelpful illness beliefs' about what they could or couldn't do. Under this regime, many relapsed. Today the view is that people with CFS should combine rest with gentle activity on the days when they feel well enough. Perhaps if I explain my own story, you can see how yoga can be effective in fulfilling the so-called 'activity' criteria.

In 1992 I was hospitalised with severe CFS. Part of my treatment was graded exercise. My experience of this was mixed. On the one hand, it helped me to get physically stronger and develop muscle strength, which meant that I could walk again. On the other, on days when I exercised, I simply had no energy left for anything else and sometimes I felt much worse. I was lucky; I worked with an understanding physiotherapist who didn't push me. If I relapsed, I was allowed to bed-rest until I felt stronger. Physiotherapists who are not flexible in this are at risk of pushing their patients into further ill health. When I came out of hospital, I joined a remedial yoga class, which was brilliant because it allowed me to work within my own boundaries. Nobody ever pushed me to do more, and if I was too ill to attend a class, I could usually do a few stretches at home. This then helped my health to steadily improve.

My personal view is that those of us with CFS need to attempt some kind of activity within our boundaries, but the old-fashioned view of rigid graded exercises is unhelpful. Graded exercise programmes only work if they are flexible and take account of the individual's fluctuations. Graded exercises can be harmful for some if the practitioner has not recognised the physical limitation of CFS and assumes the illness is due to deconditioning because of 'illness beliefs'. Practitioners should always listen to their patients, rather than pushing them to the point at which they 'crash'. I think a quote from Dr Mason Brown, who has recovered from CFS himself, sums up the situation on graded exercises quite well: 'Being scientifically logical, would any doctor treat a patient with angina of their heart with only graded exercise...? No. Then, why in ME with recurrent decreased brain and pituitary circulation, treat it with only graded exercise...? It is illogical.' Dr Brown goes on to explain that exercise has to be appropriate to the patient's health and paced with rest.

In a report carried out by Action for ME and the ME Association, out of over 1,000 people questioned with severe CFS, 50 per cent said that graded exercise made them worse, and only 34 per cent said it made them better. (The rest said it made no difference.) The conclusions of the survey were that, for some, complete rest is helpful, but this can include relaxation (such as the Pose of Complete Rest), as opposed to bed-rest. However, excessive rest can also be harmful, simply because muscles become deconditioned. Short walks, breathing exercises and gentle yoga are recommended by the charity for those who are well enough - but the most important feature in coping with, or overcoming, CFS is in pacing your activities. In the survey, almost all had tried pacing their activities and 90 per cent reported that this had helped them.

Action for ME advises against embarking upon graded exercises where increases in activity are imposed with no regard to the patient's reaction. Instead, they recommend that you rest in the acute stage of your illness, then experiment with the level of activity (physical and mental) that you can manage, without causing a relapse, then gradually increase this only if you don't feel any worse. The more successful graded exercise programmes now share many of the principles of those of pacing. They agree a baseline, encourage gradual improvement and recognise plateaux and relapses. Even so, the best practitioners would not claim to help more than half of those they treat and, sadly, there are still clinicians who impose rigid programmes that can make people worse rather than better.

In summary then, we can see that CFS is a very real and disabling condition which affects many of the systems in the body. This means that any activity has to be approached with caution. As we will discover in the next chapter, this is where yoga comes in.

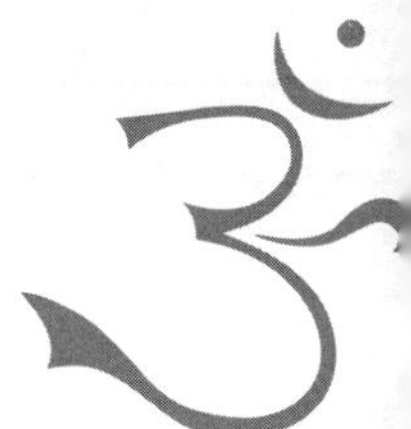

why yoga works for CFS

With any chronic illness such as CFS, it is important to maintain some mobility, if at all possible, as this can create energy and stop muscle and joint atrophy. I hope I have convinced you by now of the value of practising yoga if you have CFS. It is an activity you can do at home, which costs you nothing, and which you can practise entirely within your own limits. Also, as we have seen, CFS is a disease affecting immune, CNS, endocrine, circulation and detoxification functions. Yoga helps to normalise and regulate all of these systems. We have also seen that aerobic exercise may be harmful for CFS sufferers. However, according to Professor Cheney, the anaerobic pathway is largely intact with CFS. That means that gentle stretching, such as in yoga, can maintain muscle tone and strength and improve the elimination of toxins – without provoking a relapse. Yoga postures are of great benefit because, as well as keeping your whole system going, they also create a proper exchange of oxygen with other gases in your blood, so that your cells can burn up the food you have eaten and convert it into energy

In particular, yoga helps CFS because it:

- helps to calm the central nervous system, especially through the relaxation exercises;
- uses meditation, relaxation and visualisation exercises, which help the brain to go into an Alpha state, where brain waves slow down. This is deeply healing and an antidote to the 'fight and flight' mechanism;
- reduces stress in many ways;
- increases mental focus and helps with 'foggy head' and cognitive problems;

- helps to transport oxygen more efficiently to the cells, thereby giving you much more energy – the breathing exercises are particularly good for this;
- counteracts any problems caused by hyperventilation by teaching correct breathing control;
- helps normalise endocrine function – the postures are particularly good for this;
- helps to detoxify the system by gently stimulating your lymphatic mechanism;
- generally improves your lungs and circulation system;
- strengthens organs, bones, joints, muscles and spinal cord;
- improves digestion – irritable bowel syndrome and allergies are often common problems in CFS;
- gives you more energy, rather than using it up like normal cardiovascular exercise;
- offers the benefits of exercise, but in a gentle way that won't trigger a relapse;
- works on your chakras, or energy centres;
- may introduce you to the spiritual philosophy, giving a more positive meaning to your life.

The beauty of yoga is that you can practise it at any level – without ever overdoing it – as one of the principles of yoga is listening to your body and keeping within your limits. So, if you have severe CFS, you can do breathing and relaxation exercises – and maybe, on a good day, some gentle stretches. Whatever you do however, you need to listen to your body and be aware of your limits. It's the law of diminishing returns – you reach a point at which you gain maximum benefit from yoga. Push yourself any further and you could trigger a relapse. You have to decide what that point is, and never be tempted to cross it.

Remember to Pace Yourself

When considering any form of exercise, the idea of 'limit setting' or pacing yourself, as we saw in the last chapter, is probably the most important thing you can do. Professor Cheney says about activity in general: 'Find the boundaries of what you can do and then stay within them. Both trying to do too much, and doing too little are counter-productive. People with CFS are very susceptible to the push-crash phenomena and you need to stay within certain boundaries. To the extent you do that, you will tend to do better.' In other words, yoga will make you better, providing you don't over-do things.

Listen to Your Body and Set Your Limits

So, remember – you can do yoga postures at your own rate, according to your level of health. There is *no* competition, so you don't have to push yourself into relapse. The first step is learning to listen to your body so that you can take note of how you feel and pace yourself on that particular day. Work out your own yoga programme, using the guide below. You may start with just breathing, stretching or meditation. Always do less than you think you can do. For example, if you feel well enough to do 20 minutes of yoga postures, do only 10 minutes – and if you think you can do 10, just do five. Five minutes a day is better than no minutes and is a base on which to build. Aim to work slowly, to add perhaps an extra posture every month. Don't be tempted to do too much on a good day. If you are having a bad day, or a relapse, or are very ill, then just practise the relaxation and breathing exercises. People with CFS tend to be perfectionists – we want to be the best. But think of your yoga practice as learning that you don't need to think like this any more. Your best is what you can manage, and no more. As long as you build up your muscle tolerance slowly, set yourself small, achievable goals, pace yourself, keep to your limits and are patient, you will find that gentle yoga helps tremendously. The road back to good health will be long and slow – but yoga will take you in the right direction.

If you have mild or moderate CFS, you may be able to do more, perhaps even join a class. A word of warning – do find the right teacher. Iyengar or Ashtanga yoga, for example, will be too dynamic for most people with CFS and could put you off yoga for life! All the yoga in this book is based on classical yoga. I would, however, advise you not to join an ordinary yoga class until you have made considerable progress in your recovery; it is too easy to overdo things and relapse. Either join a remedial class or follow the postures in this book that you feel well enough to do at home. Angela Stevens (see Useful Addresses) has a list of yoga teachers who specialise in teaching CFS sufferers in the UK.

How to Approach Your Yoga Practice

- Set yourself a programme of rest and activity times throughout the day. Include in this one gentle session of yoga, according to your level of health.
- Remember that mental activities count as well as physical ones.
- When your energy levels are good, take advantage of this, but do *not* push yourself beyond your limits.
- Find your baseline – how much yoga you can do – and don't cross this for several weeks, until you are confident in adding a few more stretches.
- On a good day, do not be tempted to do too much. Remember, CFS fluctuates, so don't go mad! Pacing is about discovering your limitations and learning how much you can do, without triggering a relapse.
- Remember – yoga is not just about doing physical postures. Relaxation, breathing exercises, visualisations and meditation are all part of yoga, so on a day when you feel physically drained, you can still do some yoga practice.

You need to learn to tune yourself in – to be aware of the difference between a 'healthy' tiredness and the 'unhealthy', poisoned feeling you get after too much activity, or if you have pushed yourself too far. Listen to your body. Remember that a relapse from overdoing things can occur up to three days after activity. Also, please remember that we are all individuals. I am not with you, and even if I were, I am not in your head, so to speak, so I can't understand your particular health restrictions. Only you can work this out for yourself, so you need to be very clear in how much activity you do. To help you, I am going to describe Professor Findley's parameters of CFS, so that you can decide which category you fit into, and then be guided by how much yoga you do according to that.

The Different Levels of CFS

Professor Findley, a neurologist, who runs an ME clinic in the UK, categorises ME (his term for CFS) into the following:

Mild ME – Sufferers are mobile and can take care of themselves, doing light domestic tasks. They may be able to work, but to do so, will have stopped all leisure and social activities, often using the weekend to rest.

Moderate ME - These are people who have reduced mobility and are restricted in all activities of daily living, often having peaks and troughs during the day. They usually cannot work and require rest periods, often sleeping in the afternoon. Sleep quality in general is poor.

Severe ME - This group can only carry out minimal tasks such as brushing teeth. They have severe cognitive difficulties and will be wheelchair bound. They are usually unable to leave the house and will have severe after-effects from any effort.

Very Severe ME - Sufferers are not mobile, cannot carry out any task for themselves and are in bed for most of the time. They cannot tolerate noise or bright light.

Clearly then, ME or CFS affects all of us in different ways - from those who can have a reasonable quality of life, through to those who are completely disabled and crippled by this illness.

In the following sections, I am going to use Professor Findley's categories and recommend a yoga programme for each one. From this, you can select the yoga routine that you think will work best for you, but please bear in mind your own individual response and fluctuations - and always start by doing less than you think you can do before you build up. Also, you can 'pick and mix' from the different categories, depending on how your health varies. What you will find, over a period of time, is that if you can practise a little bit of yoga every day, then your health will start to improve and you will have much more energy. Remember to always start and finish with a five-minute relaxation posture, such as the Pose of Complete Rest.

Mild CFS

If you haven't done any yoga before, you may like to try the postures listed under Moderate CFS first, to see how you react. You may also like to try the yoga DVD I have made with another teacher to go with this book (see Useful Addresses). If you are fine with these, then an excellent programme to try is called 'The Rishikesh Sequence', a classical set of gentle postures that provide a complete workout. I have modified this for those of you who have not done yoga before, to make it slightly easier. For example, I have replaced the Full Shoulder Stand with the Half Shoulder Stand, the Pose of Tranquillity has replaced the Plough and the Cobra takes the place of the Sphinx.

Modified Rishikesh Sequence for CFS

This combines forward, backward, rotating and twisting sequences, which work to counterpose each other for complete harmony. It also includes an inverted position - excellent for energy.

Start by doing a few warm-up stretches. Lie down on your back, in a straight line. Relax your breathing. Lie in the relaxation pose.

Half Shoulder Stand - Lie on your back with your arms by your sides and your palms down. Relax. Now, breathing in, swing your legs and trunk into the air, bringing your hips off the ground. Immediately support your hips with your hands so that your legs and hips are at an angle of about 45 degrees to your trunk. Hold this position, keeping your neck and shoulders relaxed, and breathe normally for about a minute, from your ribcage. Relax into the posture. Let your hands support your back, keeping your little fingers as close together as possible.

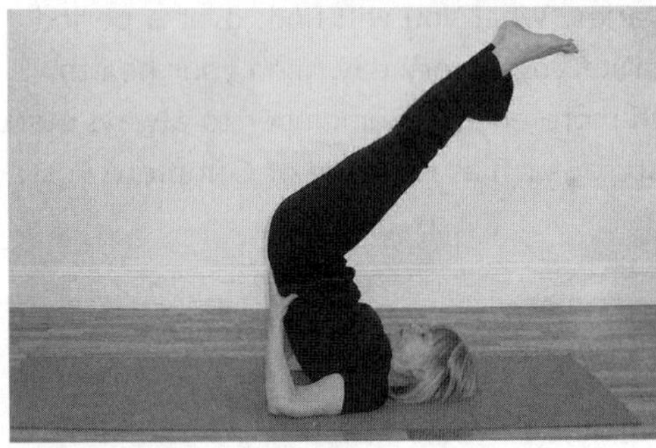

Half Shoulder Stand

Pose of Tranquillity (optional) - From the Half Shoulder Stand, work your body upwards, so that your spine and legs are straight and you are resting on your shoulders. Next, start to lower your legs behind your head, without bending them, so that they are at an angle of about 45 degrees to the floor. You should feel a point of balance somewhere between the base of your neck and your shoulder blades. When you feel balanced, bring up your arms and hold your ankles or shins. Hold for about 30 seconds. Keep your eyes closed and breathe normally. To come out of this posture, breathe out and slowly bring your knees towards your chest. Arch your neck to keep your head down and roll your spine and hips down slowly onto the floor. Rest.

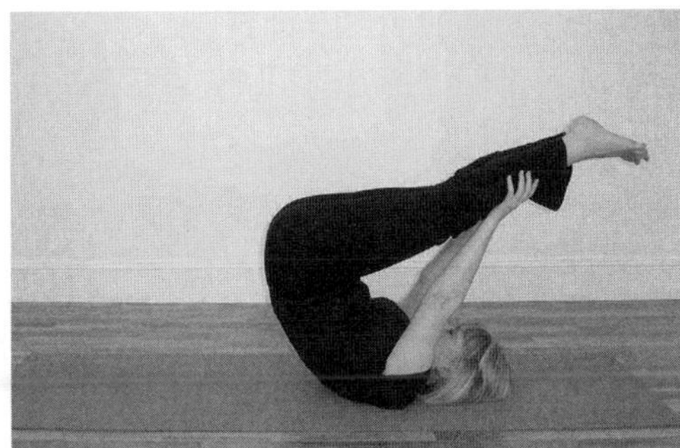

Pose of Tranquillity

The Fish - From the relaxation pose, take your arms under your body, so that you are lying on them, with your hands under your hips and your shoulders pulled down. Pushing on your elbows, gently lift your chest and shoulders from the floor, so that your neck is free and your head is lifted. Carefully take your head down towards the floor, relaxing your neck. Gently rest on the back of your head, but with your elbows taking most of your weight. Your chest should be lifted. Stay like this for about 15 seconds to counterpose the Half Shoulder Stand. Now relax your head back onto the floor and take your arms back to your sides. Rest. Roll your head from side to side to release any tension.

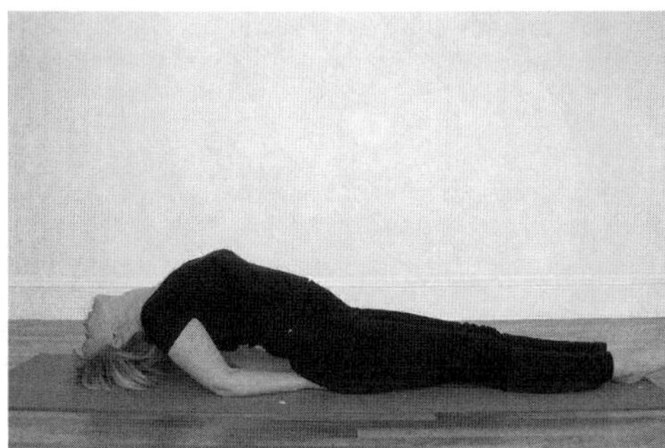

The Fish

Sitting Forward Stretch - From your relaxation posture, breathe in, then take your arms back over your head on an out-breath. Now breathe in, swing your arms forward and sit up, with your legs in front of you. On the next in-breath, take both arms and stretch up towards the ceiling. On the next out-breath, hinge forward from your hips, keeping your back straight, and fold your chest towards your thighs. Rest your arms on your legs. On each out-breath, try to come slightly more forward, towards your thighs, but without bending your back. Hold as long as is comfortable. Now breathe in, come up and relax back onto the floor. Sit up and repeat once more. Relax again. As you relax, visualise life force and energy travelling up through your feet, coming up towards the top of your head. Imagine this in waves of energy, passing through you.

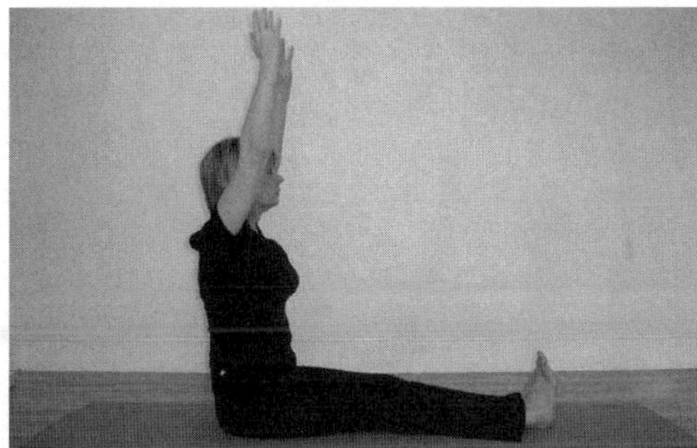

Reaching up to sitting stretch

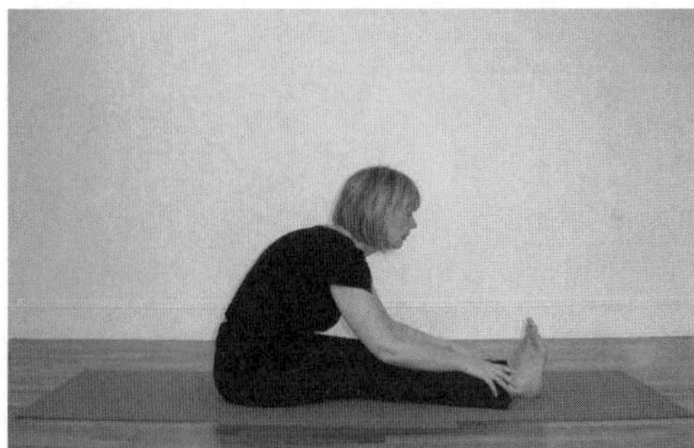

Reaching further forward

Backward Bend - Sphinx – Roll onto your front. Have your head on one side and arms by your side, with your palms uppermost. Now lift the upper half of your body, resting on your forearms and hands, making sure that your elbows are directly under your shoulders. Pull your shoulders back towards your feet and lift the crown of your head towards the ceiling, so that your breastbone is in a vertical position. Keep your shoulders soft and your elbows bent, so that your arms form a square shape. Don't slump. Look straight ahead and hold for a few seconds, visualising white energy pouring into the base of your spine and filling your body. Come down slowly on an out-breath, and relax on the floor with your head to the other side.

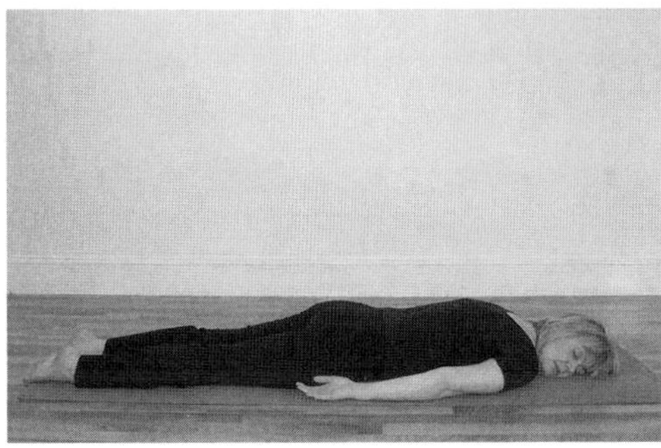

Lying on front

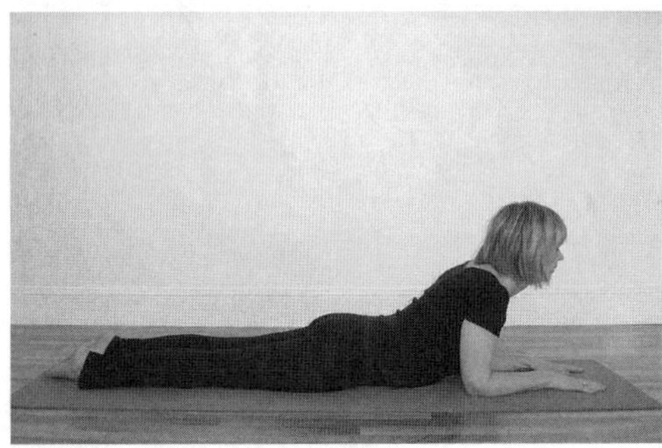

Sphinx

Half Locust - Put your chin onto the floor. Bring your feet together. Make fists with your hands and take your hands under your hips. This will give you leverage for the next movement. Now, on an in-breath, lift your right leg, keeping contact with your hips on your fists. Hold for a few seconds, keeping your leg straight. On an out-breath, lower your leg slowly back to the floor. Repeat on the left side, then repeat once more on each side. Remember to keep your chin on the floor and your pelvis level. Relax, with your head on the other side from which you had it before.

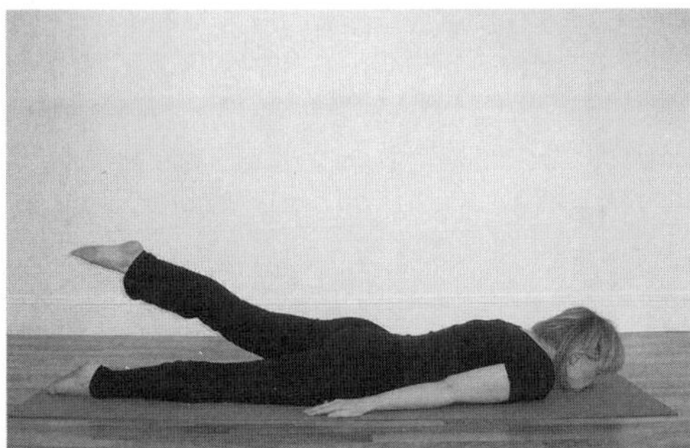

Half Locust

Full Locust (optional) - As before, keep your chin on your chest, but this time, breathe in and lift both legs together. Don't lift your hips from your fists. Lower your legs slowly as you breathe out and relax. Don't hold the position for too long. Repeat, if you are not too tired. This is a much stronger position – so only do this if you have practised yoga before and your CFS really is very mild!

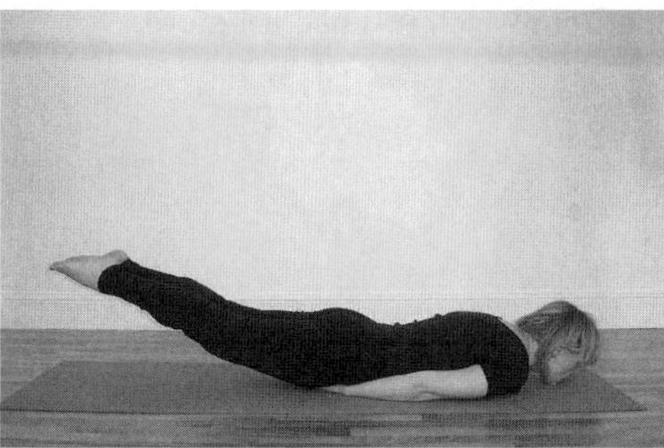

Full Locust

Now roll onto your back, hug your knees to your chest and rock from side to side. Lift your head to your knees. Sit up.

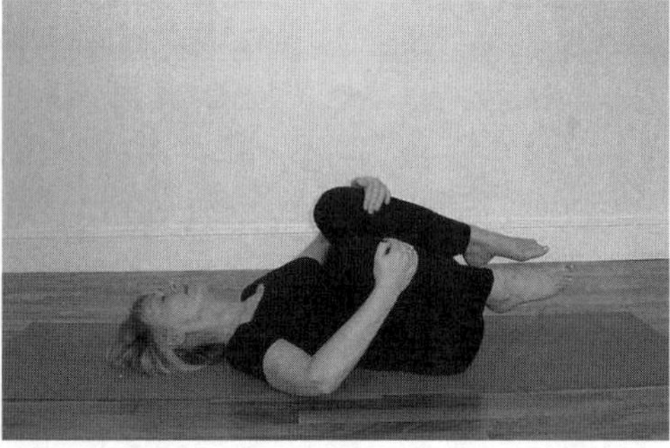

Rocking from side to side

Spinal Twist - Have your legs straight in front of you. Sit up straight - don't slump. Bring your right leg over your left leg and place your foot level with the outside of your left knee. Squeeze the right knee into the elbow of the left arm. Raise the right arm to shoulder level, hand and arm parallel to the floor, then sweep the arm around to the right, dropping the fingers behind the spine. Turn your head to look over your right shoulder. Work upwards from the base of your spine so that as you make the movement, your spine lengthens and the right side of your abdomen lifts, followed by your ribs and chest. Sit upright as you rotate your body.

Note - if you don't like the sitting Spinal Twist, you can replace it with the lying-down Crocodile Twist (see page 127).

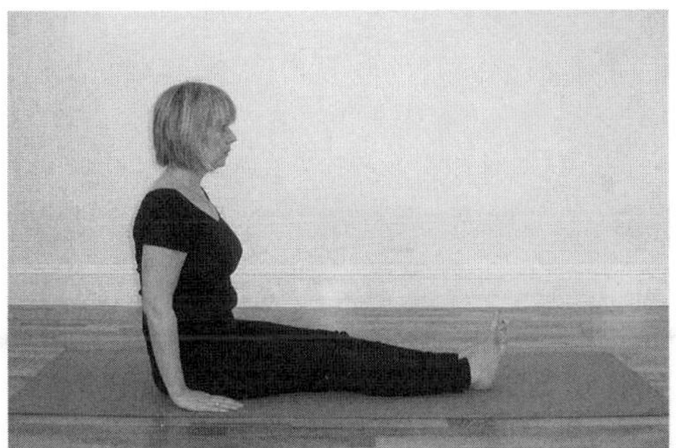

Sitting up

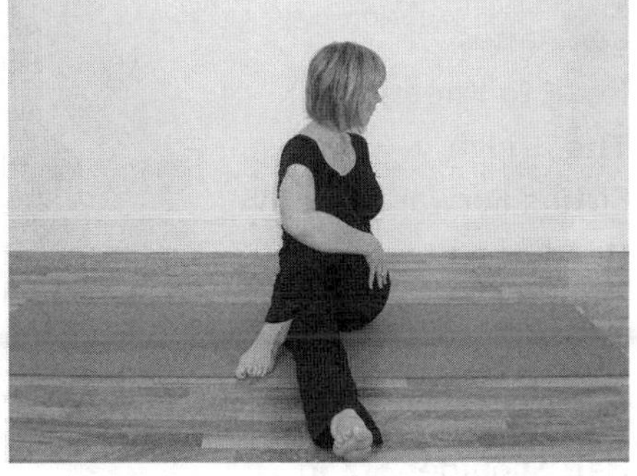

Spinal Twist

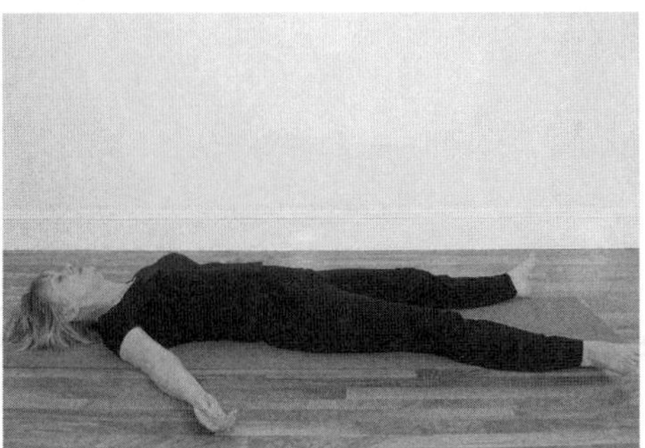

Pose of Complete Rest

Moderate CFS

Below, I have listed a two-day sequence of postures that you can try at home. Experiment. If this is too much, then leave out some of the poses. You will find all the descriptions of the postures in Chapters 5-8.

Day One

Pose of Complete Rest
Lying Down Stretch (warm up)
The Crocodile Twist
Leg Raises
Head to Knee Pose
The Bridge
Sitting Forward Stretch
Head of a Cow
Shoulder Shrugs
Neck Roll
The Lion
Half Shoulder Stand
The Butterfly
The Fish
Pose of Complete Rest

Day Two

Remember that you can select from these poses. If you find any of them too hard or too simple, then make up your own routine. For day two, I have included some gentle standing stretches for those of you well enough to do these.

Pose of Complete Rest
Lying Down Stretch
Leg Raises

The Butterfly
The Mountain Pose
Sideways Bend

The Modified Tree For this, simply stand on one leg and bend the other leg behind you, holding your ankle. Alternatively, you may like to just bend your knee and lift your foot slightly up from the ground. Hold your hands in a prayer position, over your chest.

The Holy Fig Tree Stand in the Mountain Pose. Stretch your right arm up to the ceiling and your left hand out to the side and parallel to the floor, stretching out towards the wall. Now take your left leg and point it behind you, touching the floor. If you feel confident, lift your foot slightly from the floor, so that you are stretching in a three-way direction. Hold for about 30 seconds, and then change sides. This is an exceptionally energising posture.

Standing Forward Stretch
The Sphinx
The Cat
Half Shoulder Stand
Pose of Complete Rest
Alternate Nostril Breathing

Severe CFS

Depending on how severe your CFS is, you may like to try some simple joint rotations and stretches. Lie on top of your bed to do these, or sit on the bed if necessary. You should focus your yoga practice on relaxation, pranayama (breathing exercises, see Chapter 4) and meditation, which is explained in the next chapter. It will be very beneficial to your system if you can do some of the stretches - but only do what you can and don't push yourself. Refer to Chapters 5-7 for instructions.

Daily Routine

Pose of Complete Rest
Pigeon Hole visualisation

Basic Breathing Lie down, with your eyes closed, and breathe slowly and rhythmically from your diaphragm. Notice the difference between your out-breath and your in-breath. Now, for one minute, breathe in for a count of four, and out for a count of six. Then return to normal breathing. As you breathe in, visualise calmness and energy flooding your whole body. As you breathe out, imagine all negativity and illness being blown away.

Leg Raises These may be too much for you – but they will help to strengthen your hamstring muscles, which will help you with walking and standing. If you can, lie on your bed, bend your right knee towards your chest, then straighten your leg and point your toe towards the ceiling. Rotate your foot first one way for a minute, then the other way. Do the same with your left leg. Practise this every other day, increasing the time you hold your leg. If you can't do this, remember do *not* push yourself.

Full Body Stretch Wriggle down to the centre of your bed. Clasp your hands together and take your arms behind your head and stretch them towards the wall. At the same time, point your toes and stretch your legs. Release the stretch, and then repeat, this time flexing your heels. Repeat twice. Try to time this movement with your breath, so that you breathe in to stretch and out as you relax.

Now, if you can, sit up on your bed. From sitting:

Windmill
Neck Roll
Shoulder Shrug
Joint exercises
The Lion

Inverted posture (Get onto the floor, lie down with your feet on the bed, so that your legs are raised. Relax for several minutes.)

Pose of Complete Rest
Alternate Nostril Breathing

The above sequence is designed to stretch your body and mobilise your joints, whilst calming your system down using relaxation and yoga breathing. Do progress to meditation if you feel well enough – you will find it very helpful.

Very Severe CFS

I am very aware that severe CFS is totally disabling. Therefore I am not including any physical yoga. You can try any of the breathing exercises in the book (except Kapalabhati), and attempt the visualisations and meditation exercises. If you are able, gentle stretching will help you. From your wheelchair, simply link your hands together and stretch them out in front of you. Then try lifting one leg at a time, keeping it straight and holding for a couple of seconds. If you can, lie on the bed or floor with your legs raised on some cushions or pillows so that your legs are higher than your heart. Stay like this for at least five minutes, to encourage blood-flow towards your head. This will give you similar benefits to an inverted posture.

The exercise below is called 'Yoga nidra' which is one of the most effective ways I know of completely calming the mind. It will also help to relax your central nervous system, which will benefit your CFS. Yoga nidra means 'sleep' but it involves a state of relaxation while you are conscious, which is claimed to be as effective as eight hours of normal sleep. At the same time, you remain fully in control and can come out of the relaxation at any time.

Yoga nidra uses a set of instructions, which quickly rotate the attention around the body and this simply induces a very deep sense of relaxation and wellbeing. If you find it difficult to concentrate or focus, then just let the words drift over you. I suggest you get someone who has a pleasant voice to read this out to you (perhaps your carer) or record it onto an audiotape, so that you can listen as you lie down with your eyes closed. If you would like more yoga nidra tapes, a good selection is available from Angela Thompson's tapes and books, telephone (UK) 0208 599 6781. Alternatively, Angela Stevens has produced an audiotape especially for those confined to bed called *Energise and Relax with Yoga*. This focuses on breathing, visualisation and the chakras. It is an excellent tape, one I can thoroughly recommend. (See Useful Addresses for further details.)

Yoga Nidra

Lie comfortably on your bed and relax as much as possible. Be aware of your breathing. Notice your body and how you feel today. Feel the contact of your body on the bed. Notice where your body makes contact and where there are spaces. Try to keep still, without falling asleep. Just be aware of your whole body. Watch your breathing – don't try to change it, just be aware of it and observe it. Say to yourself, 'I am calm, I have energy, I am practising yoga nidra'. Repeat this to yourself three times. You are now going to take your mind around your body, just observing each part as it is mentioned.

Feel the thumb of your right hand, index finger, middle finger, ring finger, little finger, palm, back of the hand, whole hand, wrist, forearm, elbow, upper arm, shoulder, armpit, right side of your chest, waist, hip, thigh, knee, back of your knee, calf muscle, lower leg, ankle, heel, sole of your foot, the arch, the middle of the sole, the ball, big toe, second toe, third toe, fourth toe, little toe, experience your left hand thumb, index finger, middle finger, ring finger, little finger, your palm, back of your hand, the whole hand, wrist, forearm, elbow, upper arm, shoulder, armpit, left side of your chest, waist, hip, thigh, knee, lower leg, ankle, heel, sole, arch of the sole, ball of the foot, big toe, second toe, third toe, fourth toe, little toe. Feel both soles of your feet. Now, take your attention to your right buttock, left buttock, right side of your lower back, left side of your lower back, right side of your upper back, left side of your upper back. Right shoulder blade, left shoulder blade, spine. Your whole back, your neck, back of your head, top of your head, forehead, right temple, left temple, right ear, left ear, right cheek, left cheek, right eyebrow, left eyebrow, the space between your eyebrows. Your whole nose, the tip of your nose, tongue, lower lip, both lips, chin, throat, right chest, left chest, whole chest, heart, stomach, navel, pubic area, the whole of your right leg, whole of your left leg, whole right arm, whole left arm, the whole of your head.

Now experience your whole body. Just be aware of your whole body. Don't go to sleep. Become aware of heaviness in your whole body against the bed. Your right forearm is heavy. Now feel the weight increasing. Feel heaviness in the entire arm. Now in the left forearm, the whole arm. Your left hand, the shoulder, the whole arm. Now your head, your legs, your feet. In your abdomen and your back. Just feel heavy all over: your eyes feel heavy, your forehead and entire face feel heavy. Everything feels very heavy. Now become aware of lightness, light arms, light feet, light legs, light head and light trunk. Feel your back as weightless. Your whole body is light all over. You feel as if you could float off the bed. Now think of cold. Remember what it feels like to walk on a cold floor, to touch a cold windowpane or a snowball. Take this experience and feel cold in your whole body, as if you were lying outside in the winter. You accept this feeling – you are just observing it. Cold feet, cold hands, cold head and cold trunk. Now be aware of heat, as if you are lying on a hot beach. You just want to lie dozing in the heat as your body becomes hotter and hotter. Your hands, arms, legs, head and trunk are hot. Your navel is so warm, it pushes heat out to your whole body. Be aware but don't fall asleep. Now feel pleasure throughout your body. Imagine you are lying in your favourite place – perhaps a beautiful garden, on a beach or in the countryside. Just observe a state of carefree being. You are lying, relaxing, and feeling happy and content just to be.

Now forget your body and be aware only of your consciousness, of you, your real self who is at rest and who is just observing your physical body. Now silently repeat three times: 'I am calm, I have energy, I am practising yoga nidra'. Now start to become aware again of the contact your body is making on the bed. Notice the difference between where you are making contact on the bed and the spaces. Open your eyes. Look around the room. Do you feel any different from when you started your practice? Rub your hands together vigorously and just be aware that you are in the room.

This concludes your yoga nidra practice – you should now feel calm and deeply refreshed. I am now going to finish by giving you a true story about someone I know who has used yoga to help her to recover from CFS.

Cindy's Story

I first became ill with CFS in 1995. Up until that point I had been very healthy - I worked as a tennis coach. In the winter of 1995 I had a series of infections that I couldn't seem to shake off. I was also having marital problems, so I guess I was under stress. I just got weaker and weaker. I was sleeping all the time, and any physical or mental effort left me feeling completely drained. I had to give up work, which broke my heart. Even seeing friends became too exhausting for me. They would think I looked fine, not knowing that it then took me days to recover from any social occasion. I was in despair about my physical lack of strength; as an athlete I knew the importance of exercise but it was just impossible for me even to walk very far.

In 1997, someone recommended I visit the Yoga for Health Foundation. By this time I was in a wheelchair. I signed up for the Yoga and ME course. I was quite anxious about going because I was so ill, and was scared it would make me worse, like the graded exercise programmes I had heard about. But they were amazing to me there. The yoga teachers helped to carry me and lay me on a mat and I started with very simple routines. If I didn't feel well enough, then I stayed in bed. I was so impressed that I started a yoga class when I returned home.

At first, all I could do was sit on a chair during the class and join in with a few exercises now and again and then do the relaxation at the end. There was no pressure to push myself or to do anything I didn't feel ready for - quite the opposite in fact. Gradually, I felt I could do more and more, and after about six months, I abandoned the chair and joined in with the rest of the class, albeit in a fairly limited way. I would do one repetition of a pose where the others would do three, and I would miss out on the stronger postures altogether. By the end of the year, I was more or less able to do the whole class. Now, three years later, I am doing an hour of yoga every day at home as well as the weekly class, and I can't overstate the difference it has made to my life. People tell me that I look healthy for the first time in years, and I am able to stay awake for more of the day. I can also manage on eight hours' sleep at night - if I rest for an hour after lunch - whereas at one point I was sleeping for 14 hours a day. My bad days are fewer and further between, and they are not as intense as they used to be. On good days I feel almost back to normal, though I sometimes have a fuzzy head and can't walk for more than 40 minutes even at my best. Still, this is such an improvement!

Yoga was the only thing that worked. The yoga diet I followed has really helped me too. I just feel calmer; have more energy and I feel as if I am back in control of my body again. It struck me how different yoga was to any sport, or to what I expected. Nobody pushed me, and contrary to what people think, I didn't have to get into any funny positions! I think the breathing, relaxation and meditation particularly helped. I have now gone from having severe CFS to mild CFS. I can't teach tennis any more - but I can play the odd game. Sometimes I even win! The point for me is that yoga has given me a different perspective on my life. I am not worried about defining myself by what I do - but by who I am. It is so true that yoga teaches us the importance of being, not doing - and I think this is a vital lesson for anyone with CFS. I don't measure my worth by my accomplishments any more. I am now calmer, more centred and much happier. I have confidence and self-esteem and I put that down to learning about the philosophy behind yoga. Yoga really put me on the path back to health and I would recommend that anyone with CFS tries yoga - it has made such a huge difference to the quality of my life.

So, to conclude, I know of literally hundreds of people with CFS who have dramatically improved their health with yoga - including myself! Cindy is a very typical example and I hope, however severe your CFS, that it will inspire you to try yoga for yourself. In the next chapter, we will look at meditation. This is perhaps one of the most important aspects of yoga to concentrate on if you really want to beat fatigue or are interested in finding a spiritual dimension to your life.

11 beat fatigue with meditation

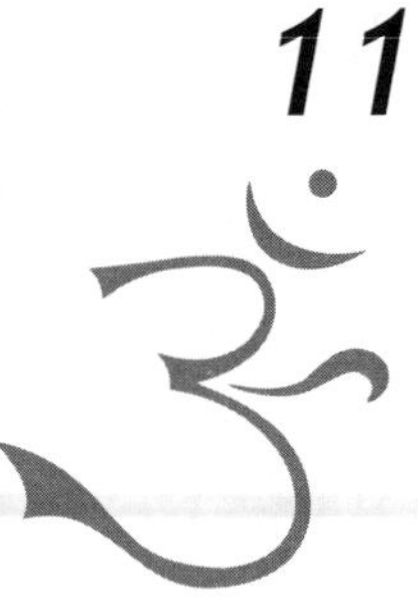

If you meditate every day, you are going to have more energy, vigour and stamina. But there are other reasons why you should meditate – these are just the 'side-effects' of meditation, an additional bonus. In Chapter 2, I explained that there are eight limbs of yoga: different elements that include the yoga postures and yoga breathing. Meditation, the seventh limb, is about finding your real self and your real truth. If you are not interested in doing this, that's fine, but you will benefit in lots of other ways because meditation can:

- calm your mind
- help you to feel relaxed
- relieve anxiety and help to take away worries
- relieve insomnia
- slow down the production of stress-related chemicals, your breathing and heart-rate
- give stamina and raise energies
- heal
- reduce information overload in the brain and give you some space
- help to bring your mind under control so that your thoughts and emotions do not sweep you along
- help you to feel more centred and balanced
- bring peace and a sense of purpose to your life
- help you to find your own truth and to get in touch with your real self.

This is quite a long list of benefits, and even if you are interested in only some of them, you can perhaps see why meditation is so popular today. However, unless you are very lucky, meditation is not usually something that just happens, or that you just 'do'. It's not just a case of clearing your mind and not thinking for 20 minutes. In fact, if you try to do this you will probably find it impossible - your mind will start buzzing with thoughts and ideas. Meditation requires practice and discipline. Later in this chapter I shall give you some guidelines on how to start meditating. In the meantime, I'm going to explain a bit more about the mind and why meditation can help you.

Meditation is said to take place when everything stops. It is the stopping - stilling your mind and listening in to silence - that is difficult. Meditation is about being able to let go of your thoughts - not by forcing them out or trying to drive them away, but by allowing them to come and go without getting involved in them. Let's think about this for a moment. It is the nature of the mind always to be active, flitting from one thing to another. This is incredibly exhausting because you are dissipating prana or vital energy as you move from one thought to another in a split second in your busy and noisy mind. Your mind loves being active; it is rather like a runaway chariot, with your thoughts being the out-of-control horses running in all directions, and you as the charioteer trying to rein them in. In this way, you may find that you are swept along in life by your emotions. As I said in Chapter 2, yoga and meditation are about control of the thought waves of your mind. Think about how one thought triggers another, then another and another, like a chain. In yoga it is believed that this thought-chain, or unruly mind, is the root of all trouble and disease - and, of course, exhaustion. The first step in meditation is to be aware of your busy mind and this chain, so that you can learn to let it go and not become involved in it. In this way meditation will help you to bring all your scattered energy back to one point.

Meditation is also about exploring your real self so that you can learn to put aside your everyday thoughts and desires. It's a bit like peeling back the layers of an onion skin to find out who you really are. As you start meditating, you may well find that it feels rather like coming home, as if you are coming back to something you are very familiar with. If you continue to meditate regularly, you will feel a sense of deep calm, relaxation and peace. This is because in your everyday activities and thinking, your brainwaves occur in spiky, fast Theta waves. When you meditate, these brainwaves change to the slower Alpha waves associated with relaxation. Eventually, you may experience even slower Delta waves, similar to those in sleep, which indicate a very deep level of relaxation. This, of course, is very restful, and as a consequence your energy will be boosted at the end of your session.

How to Meditate

You may be surprised to realise that there already is an element of meditation in your life. For example, if you are really concentrating on reading a book, driving your car or doing anything that involves your mind in a disciplined way so that it doesn't wander off into the 'chain' of thinking I mentioned earlier, you are laying the foundation for learning to meditate. If you are doing an activity such as yoga postures, gardening, painting, listening to music, walking in the countryside or watching a beautiful sunset, try and rein in your mind so that it is engrossed in just this one activity. To get the idea of this, really focus on your everyday tasks and try not to flit from one thing to another. Think only about what you are doing and really absorb yourself in the present moment without fantasising or worrying about anything else. In this way you are learning to concentrate and not wasting energy on superfluous thinking.

Preparation

To start meditating, you need to do the following:

- Find a quiet place where you will not be interrupted. The room should be warm and you should meditate in the same place at the same time every day so that you create a routine.
- Do not meditate for at least two hours after a meal, or if you are sleepy.
- The best time to meditate is first thing in the morning, at noon, or at sunset.
- If possible, sit with your spine upright, because you are working with vertical energies. If for any reason you cannot do this, lie down.
- Sit comfortably, either on a chair with your feet on the floor, or on the floor cross-legged or in the Half Lotus position.

- Hold your hands palms upwards, with your forefinger and thumb touching – or place them on your knees.
- Do not try to meditate after frenzied activity – you won't succeed! Try doing some yoga postures or yoga breathing first.
- Aim to put all your cares and worries aside for the duration of your meditation. This is your time and you don't need to think about anything else. Use the Pigeon Hole visualisation explained in Chapter 5 if you find this helpful.
- Breathe rhythmically and slowly from your diaphragm.
- You may like to imagine a white light surrounding and protecting you during your session.
- Try to close off your senses. Ignore any outside stimulation and any outside sounds you may hear. Try and turn your attention inwards. Look, with your eyes closed, at the point between your eyebrows.
- Focus on a single point, such as the rhythm of your breath.
- Meditate for 10 minutes a day at first, then gradually increase this time to 20 minutes.
- When you have finished you need to ground yourself. Never come out of meditation suddenly. Stay where you are. Wriggle your spine into your chair or onto the floor. Shake your hands. Slowly stretch your limbs.
- Finally, meditation needs both intention and effort; it isn't something that just happens. It may take you weeks, months or even longer to see the benefits, so practise, practise, practise. The results will be well worth the effort.

Different Ways to Meditate

Creative Meditation

Creative meditation is an excellent way to start. It involves thinking about one word, which you can then build on within the boundaries of that concept. For example, you take an idea or theme such as Love, Peace, Harmony, Health, God or Energy, which you then hold in your mind. You continue by thinking only about words relating to this theme during your practice. You should use only constructive or positive words so that your energies are led upwards – destructive or selfish thinking will lead to fear, anxiety and exhaustion.

Exercise

Select one of the words I suggested above. Now sit quietly for 10 minutes with your eyes closed and concentrate on this word or things associated with this word. In this way you can build up ideas from your chosen word. For example, if you chose the word Love you may think of joy, happiness, your family, and so on. The difficult thing is to keep focused on your chosen theme, building up ideas on the word but not letting your mind wander to other ideas away from your chosen theme. This isn't easy, I know, but don't give up! If your mind starts to wander; bring it back gently to ideas about the word you have chosen. Don't try to force your mind; if unrelated thoughts enter your mind, just observe them and let them go without becoming involved in their chain. Don't get frustrated if you find this difficult.

Now review what happened. Did you feel uncomfortable? Did outside sounds disturb you? Did your mind wander off? If it did, don't be disheartened; keep practising and eventually you will find that your mind starts to become stiller, which in turn will give you a deep sense of calm and more energy.

Concentration

Concentration is said to be the brickwork of meditation. It is about keeping your mind focused on only one thing, so that it is one-pointed and not dissipated. If you can focus on just one seed, such as a word or image, you can start to still your mind and turn your attention inwards, which leads on to meditation. I mentioned earlier that it will help if you live your life by focusing on the present moment and not jumping from one pursuit to another. This in turn will help your concentration. Using the analogy of a wheel, I can explain better by saying that if you live your life on the rim, you will rush about from one experience to the next, trying to find happiness and contentment. However, if you return to the still, peaceful centre of the wheel, you will find that this contentment comes from inside yourself, rather than from the pursuit of external objects. By turning your concentration and your attention inwards, you focus your mind on your inner world, where you will find a state of peace whatever happens to you. Concentration and meditation will take you away from activities which involve disturbance, confusion and restlessness. This is why meditation can give you energy.

Concentration is not as easy as it sounds, but when learning to meditate it usually takes the form of following the breath, or concentrating on an image or word. Or you can use a mantra; a sound with meaning.

Exercises

You may like to try all the suggestions given here for learning to concentrate, but once you have found one that suits you I suggest you stick to it and use the same method every day.

1 Using your breath is a powerful way to achieve concentration. Sit quietly with your eyes closed for 10 minutes. Start by focusing on the natural rhythm of your breathing. Observe it but don't force it; just let it happen naturally. You can try any of the following:
   - Concentrating on your breathing, count mentally from one to four on each in-breath. If your mind wanders and you forget to count, bring your attention back to the natural rhythm of your breath and start at one again.
   - Just watch your breath, focusing on the feeling as it comes in and out of your nostrils. Feel how it is cool as you breathe in and warmer as you exhale. Notice any sibilant sound it makes. Watch the rise and fall of your diaphragm. Focus on the space between your breaths. Notice the stillness. Hear the silence.
   - You can use the traditional Ham Sa breathing mantra. Mentally say 'Ham' as you breathe in and 'Sa' as you breathe out. Ham Sa is called the natural mantra because it's repeated by every living thing that breathes.

2 A mantra (a single word or short phrase) is another powerful tool for concentration. The sound and vibration of a mantra channel energy and help the mind to become focused. Traditional mantras are carefully constructed to purify and transform.

   Om, which is said to be the sound of the whole universe, is one of the best mantras to start with. It is beneficial at a very profound level if practised every day and can bring about changes in your life quite rapidly, because it helps you to tune into your real self. Om is also very balancing; it massages the vital organs, increases blood flow, stimulates the nervous system and relaxes the respiratory system (see Chapter 3).

Another traditional mantra you may like to try is 'Om mani padme hum'. This means the 'Jewel in the Heart of the Lotus', but the vibration and rhythm of the words are just as effective as their meaning.

You can choose your own mantra, but whatever word or phrase you use, immerse yourself in the sound and become absorbed in it. You can say it out loud or silently, in time with your breath.

3 You can concentrate on an object such as a candle flame, a flower or a roaring fire. Or you may like to pick an image that has significance for you, such as the Cross, the Buddha or the Om symbol (see below). Having studied your chosen object, close your eyes and focus on it with your mind's eye for 10 minutes. If your attention wanders, open your eyes, look at the object, then close them again.

4 Yoga postures can be a form of meditation in themselves. When you hold a yoga posture and focus only on that, your mind is kept within the boundaries of the task in hand and will start to become still. This is why yoga is often called action in inaction. So if you want to prepare for meditation, you can make a start by concentrating on each yoga position as you hold it, without allowing your mind to wander.

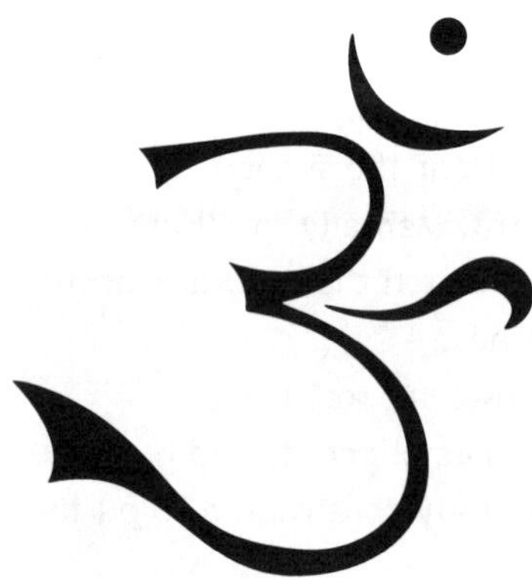

Om symbol

Receptive Meditation

If you have practised the above exercises for some time, you may now like to try stilling your mind. By this I don't mean that you should empty your mind but, rather, that you observe your thoughts without getting involved in them, and without following the 'thought chain'. If you try to push your thoughts away too hard you will give them energy; so please don't worry if you find this difficult. It takes time and perseverance to still your mind. When you meditate you lose thoughts of 'I' or 'mine' - and this is something you can't force. It may take weeks or months, or it may just happen!

Exercises

1 Sit quietly for 10-20 minutes with your eyes closed, as described earlier under Preparation. Think of your mind as a calm pool, with no ripples. If thoughts occur, observe them and let them go, but don't become involved. If your attention wanders, bring it back by listening to the silence between your breaths.

2 Visualise a stormy sea gradually calming down until it becomes smooth and quiet. The sea is your mind, and as it becomes quiet, listen to the vibrant presence of the silence. Keep your awareness in the present moment so that your thoughts are neither suppressed nor encouraged, just witnessed.

I said at the beginning of this chapter that meditation is about controlling the thought waves of the mind, and I also explained how this could then release great energy. Meditation is really about replacing the thoughts that arise from desires, restlessness and dissatisfaction with thoughts of harmony and contentment. In this way you will find not only more energy but also inner peace. Meditation will lead you back to your true nature and help you to still your mind so that you are in control.

12 my story

I'd like to finish this book by telling you something about myself, my own personal understanding of fatigue and how this brought me to yoga. Everything I've written in this book is taken from my own experience, which is why I know that yoga can beat fatigue.

I suffered from the most severe form of fatigue – ME – before yoga helped my recovery. In 1989 I was running a successful public relations company. My job was very stressful and I worked very long hours. I didn't take lunch breaks or holidays and I often worked at weekends. In order to prop up my flagging energy levels I ate lots of junk food, including sweets and chocolate. When I went home I would drink a bottle of wine to numb the exhaustion and slow down my racing brain and I would heat up a ready-prepared meal in the microwave.

The first warning I got that all was not well was panic attacks. For no apparent reason I would start to feel shaky, anxious and very strange, as if I wasn't really there. I would have difficulty getting my breath. This was followed by chronic insomnia; sometimes I went for two or three nights without sleeping at all. I thought the answer was to ignore the distress signals my body was sending me and work harder. I also joined an aerobics class, which I squeezed in to my lunch hour. The fatigue was incredible – I was always tired – but I just ignored the exhaustion and got on with running my business. In fact, I didn't really think about the fatigue – I just assumed that it was normal, that life was like that and it was something I just had to accept.

Then I got what I thought was flu. After three days in bed I dragged myself back to work. I was totally wiped out and dizzy, but I thought I had to work or my world would cave in - especially as I owed the bank £50,000 and had a huge mortgage of at least treble that amount. My doctor took some blood tests and later told me I had glandular fever caused by the Epstein-Barr virus. She advised me to rest, so I slowed down a bit - but not enough. Three months later I sold my business. I then started working as a television researcher but consequently developed some unnerving symptoms that I couldn't ignore. The exhaustion would get so bad that sometimes I couldn't even speak, and I would have to go and lie down. One day my husband found me on the floor - I couldn't move!

If I rested I was still tired. I managed to struggle on with my job, even though it meant lying down during the lunch hour rather than socialising with others in the production team. This way, I managed to keep my condition secret from my work colleagues. To admit to being tired or ill was something that wasn't allowed in our hard-driven consumer society. I existed on chocolate for a quick boost of energy but that soon wore off.

Eventually I became so ill that I had to give up work. Resting didn't make me any better and if I exercised it took me days to recover. My muscles ached. I had a permanent fog in my head and I just couldn't sleep. Eventually I was diagnosed with ME or Chronic Fatigue Syndrome. If only I had listened to my body when it had first sent me signals to slow down,

My health deteriorated until, in 1992, I was in a wheelchair. At this point I was too tired even to hold a conversation. I was also facing some prejudice, in those days some of my friends and family, encouraged my bad press and ignorant doctors were very scathing and didn't believe that I had a real physical illness. However, simple things like making a cup of tea were like climbing a mountain and if I over-exerted myself it would take days to recover. I was taken into hospital for three months and put on various drugs, which, in hindsight, made me much worse. I was also given Cognitive Behaviour Therapy. This didn't improve my energy but it did make me much more positive about life and my outlook. I also met a wonderful woman in hospital called Nancy Farley who introduced me to meditation.

In 1993 my local yoga teacher, Angela Stevens, asked me if I would help her to set up a yoga group for people with CFS. She had noticed that this was a common problem and thought that remedial yoga would help. I wasn't so sure – strenuous exercise was the last thing that I needed – but Angela assured me that yoga would be beneficial. So I got together a group of people and we started. Almost immediately I began to feel better. Angela concentrated on yoga breathing, relaxation and meditation. There were some gentle stretching exercises to get our systems going and to build up our muscle groups but we took these very slowly and at our own pace. Sometimes I over-estimated my health and did too much but that was usually because I was trying to keep up with someone on a higher level of ability. The first rule of yoga is to listen to the body and work with it, not against it! I started visiting the Yoga for Health Foundation, which was, in 1993, the largest residential yoga centre in Europe. They were doing a lot of work with ME as well as with other chronic conditions – and I learned more about the importance of proper diet and meditation During my time there studying and practising yoga, the improvement in my health became so dramatic that I realised that yoga was having a profound effect on my well -being. Pranayama – or yoga breathing – was really important in my journey back to health, as were the relaxation and stretching postures. Gradually I became physically stronger. I also became much more spiritually aware as the more I practised yoga; the more I was getting in touch with the 'real' Fiona. My teacher, Bill Feeney, says that the ego is like a large parrot on the shoulder and we should aim to reduce this to a small sparrow, in order that the ego and attachment to the material world are not driving us and that we can listen in and connect with the true inner self.

As I started to study the sutras of Patanjali in order to learn more about he philosophy of yoga. I tried to incorporate the yamas and niyamas (moral observances of conduct and restraints) in to my every day life. In studying the sutras I was also interested to learn how yoga is about controlling the mind. Since, like many people with ME I always had a hyperactive mind that used to drive me crazy and which was, no doubt, stimulating the whole of my nervous system, this touched a chord with me. Living in the present moment is a very important lesson and so the process of 'thought control', which Patanjali talks about, is, I think, vital for recovery from chronic fatigue. A mind, which is always active, is so exhausting. Staying in the here and now reduces so much tension and worry and allows us to be happy.

Also, being present helps us to be much calmer about the future. For example, if I had a relapse, I would always panic about how that would affect me, what I would have to cancel and not be able to do. This worry would then lead to further illness and exhaustion. By learning to surrender - a key lesson in yoga - I was able to just accept that this is how I was for the time being and let go of any anxieties about the future. I could choose to be ill and unhappy, or ill for now, and happy. This state of mind got me out of relapse faster than any pill I could have popped.

By 1999 I was beginning to teach yoga to other people with ME and I started a teacher training course with the Yoga for Health Foundation, which I completed in 2002. In 2003 I was contacted by Alex Howard who wanted to interview me for a CD he was making to go with his book *WHY ME?* I read Alex's book and it really resonated with me. Alex is over 20 years younger than me and yet he was giving me a lesson, which I had understood intellectually but not actually put in to action. This was that, if you want to get better, then you have to live an authentic and happy life. In other words, you have to be true to yourself and be your real self. At around the same time I read Ekhart Tolle's book *The Power Of Now*, a book I continue to refer to and which inspires me.

In 2004 I left my marriage after 24 years. My yoga journey and the lessons I learnt woke me up. I had been locked for years in an unhappy, destructive relationship which left me permanently on edge and stressed. I realised I would never truly recover until I was in a situation where I could be true to the real Fiona.
I went to work at the Yoga for Health Foundation - doing a bit of teaching but mainly working in the kitchen, which I loved. Meditation becomes so easy when doing uncomplicated tasks. In 2005 I went to do some more teaching in India and then returned to London. I was now struggling a bit emotionally as I was in the middle of a nasty divorce. I had little money and I moved to London without a job, home and without knowing many people there. I was so lucky, Martina Dodder, whom I met in India, offered me some teaching at her holistic centre in West London and a room to rent.

I then was offered more and more teaching and by the time my divorce came through I had about 15 classes a week. Considering I had been in a wheelchair ten years before I think that shows how profound the healing effect of yoga is. I am 50 now but have my independence and health and able to cope with a very physically demanding job – albeit one which I love!

All this has contributed to my recovery. I have learnt a lot more about prana since I wrote the first edition of the book. I know that, for example, when Patanjali recommended that we control our senses that, had he lived in the 21st century, he would probably advise that too much materialism, or overloading of the senses by continual TV, noise or stimulation, wears us down and takes us away from our spiritual core. I now wonder if my illness was sent to wake me up to my spiritual truth, and in that sense my ME although very traumatic, was a blessing.

People are always asking me about how to recover from ME. I would simply say: practice yoga; especially correct breathing and meditation, try to live in the present moment, eat healthy whole foods, only make constructive relationships with people who are positive and who give you pleasure and don't fritter away your energy or prana on overloading the senses with shopping, computing, radio, TV or stuff that is depleting you. Accept what is for now. And most of all, try to find your spiritual core. I sincerely hope yoga leads you to this.

postscript 13

(Or "Suffering as a Portal to Freedom")

Since the publication of '*Beat Fatigue with Yoga*' by Cherry Red books in 2006, when I wrote about my recovery from ME (Chronic Fatigue Syndrome), I have continued my journey to health. But I now realise that wellness doesn't mean something purely physical. Rather it means a true integration of peace, stability and happiness at all levels of being. To fully appreciate this though, I had to get very ill again. This is how the understanding came about.

In 2007, after teaching in London for two years, I decided to go to India. I was still hungry to know more about yoga as I felt that I wasn't getting my deeper question, 'Who am I and what is existence?', answered. I hoped that India might provide some clues. I bought a rucksack, investigated in a few ashrams (spiritual centres) on the internet, then set off. It was quite daunting, but once I was there I felt very free, and soaked up whatever I could learn. At the Vyasa ashram, near Bangalore, I studied the Bhagavad Gita, the main scriptural text of India, and learnt about the concept of karma yoga - non-attachment to the result of any action. I chanted my way around the south of the country, visiting five different ashrams and trying out various traditions of yoga. I also had an intensive bout of panchakarma - an ayurvedic detox treatment to get all the medication that I had taken when I had been ill completely out of my system. I was indulging in a kind of spiritual pick-'n-mix , but still I didn't find my answers. But I got the travel and the spiritual bug, and soon started writing for '*Yoga and Health*' magazine about my adventures.

I was full of energy and brimming with health. Next I went trekking in Nepal, then set off for Dharmasala in North India to hear teachings from the Dalai Lama and to study Tibetan Buddhism. To make ends meet and support all this seeking, I started setting up yoga retreats when I was back in the UK. Somewhat to my surprise, people with CFS and other health conditions started to come because they had read this book and were interested in trying yoga. I slowly established a network and began to specialise in teaching yoga to people with CFS and other chronic health conditions. I am completely indebted to all the many people I have worked with over the last few years – they taught me such a lot and shared their knowledge generously with me. In fact they have been my best teachers.

One of the things I learnt from these people was that there were many others like me looking for some kind of meaning in life, and also that many people with CFS had mystic experiences of oneness (sometimes called non-dual awakenings). This doesn't apply to everyone, and anyhow, experiences are nothing without understanding of their meaning, but it still seemed to me to be crucially important in 'cracking the code' and work out what Life was about – to understand the question '*What am* I?'. It seemed that, for some reason, suffering bought people closer to this.

I originally trained as a teacher with the Yoga for Health Foundation, but in 2009 I decided to do further training and become a KHYF teacher. This is the yoga tradition as taught by the great yogi Krishnamacharya, his son TKV Desikachar and now his grandson Kausthub. Based in Chennai, India, I knew that their standards were amongst the best in the world – rigorous, and of a very high quality. They maintain that yoga should be taught for the individual, and from this developed world-class training in yoga therapy. Importantly for me, there was a course in the UK which included a thorough teaching of the Yoga Sutras of Patanjali. I was blessed to have great teachers – Sarah Ryan, Liz Murtha and my mentor Gill Lloyd, whose teachings I lapped up, especially enjoying the Vedic chanting and the philosophy. What the tradition really gave me, however, was many more ways to work with my students with CFS. I learnt that the most effective tools for healing included *mantra* (sound) and *pranayama* (conscious breathing), and that yoga is about freedom – seeing through our *samskaras* (habits) to the peace of our own nature. I then started to develop teacher-training courses for yoga teachers aimed at treating fatigue and stress conditions, having realised that there was a growing need and also that there was a lot of misunderstanding around CFS/ME. Yoga could certainly help people to get better, but it could also make those with this condition worse if it wasn't taught correctly.

At the end of 2009 I attended a course on the Yoga Sutras in Chennai with Desikachar and Kausthub. I still had an idea – some kind of yearning inside – that the path of yoga, which had restored my health and energy, could lead me to understand who I was and what reality was about. The Yoga Sutras, which essentially teach a very logical and elegant psychology on how to live mindfully and how to be free by seeing reality as it is, answered some of these questions. But, like so many of us, I also had an inner voice telling me I was an inadequate being – that other people were better than me and that I needed to have the perfect relationship or job to fix this. I knew through what I had learnt about myself so far and from the study of the sutras that this wasn't actually true, but sometimes that voice nagged away at me, pushing me to try harder – pushing me to do more in order to fix myself.

After the course in Chennai, I travelled to a pilgrimage centre called Tiruvannamali, the home of the great saint Ramana Maharishi, where I intended to stay for three nights before heading further south to Kerala to spend Christmas with two friends. We even had the train tickets, but then something mysterious happened – on the second day of my stay the two friends independently had crises (the death of a relative and a stolen credit card), which meant our plans were scuppered. My friend Leah flew back to the UK, and Emma couldn't join me from Bali. I was stuck in Tiru, as it is fondly referred to, and couldn't get out of the town – every time I tried to book a ticket or make a plan, something happened to prevent me from leaving. I began to get the feeling I was meant to stay! Then I came across a notice for Vedanta teachings as taught in the Chinmayananda tradition by an American called James Swartz.

Vedanta is a traditional path of yoga known as *jnana* yoga – or the yoga of self-knowledge. It's based on the classical Indian teachings of the Bhagavad Gita, the Upanishads and the Brahma Sutras. These teachings are simply that '*I am whole and complete and need nothing outside myself to make me happy. Happiness, freedom and peace are who I am, but when I seek them in the world – through material possessions, objects or relationships – then I am bound to fail. I need to understand what is real and what isn't. That which is real is that which doesn't change – which is me*'. This knowledge, through the understanding of the teachings, leads to something known as 'self-realisation'. There is a bit more to it than this, but essentially Vedanta has a similar message to Patanjali's yoga – that we all really long for freedom and happiness and that this is our true nature. Ignorance of this causes us to feel inadequate, so we erroneously look outside of ourselves for happiness and consequently identify with the transient objects and situations around us – including our thoughts and relationships – ultimately causing ourselves to suffer. Vedanta, being a non-dual teaching, goes further and shows, through self-inquiry and understanding, that we are not really the body or mind but are pure consciousness. Through examination, questioning and contemplation, as directed by a teacher, we can understand this for ourselves and realise that there is no separation – all is one. This is known as *Advaita*, or non-duality. What I didn't know was that Tiru, this odd place that I couldn't leave, was where people came to every Winter from all over the world to 'learn about' Enlightenment.

In the end, I studied Vedanta for two years, looking at some of the main texts from the tradition and spending much time with my teacher. I also studied a little with another teacher from the Dayananda tradition, and learnt the importance of living in a way that is authentic to your nature. If you have the heart of an artist for example, and you work chasing money in business, then you may become ill from the stress of going against your nature. I learnt that the best way to live is to lead a simple and quiet life, to not be attached to the outcome of any action and not to have expectations. Without quietness and contemplation the Self is unlikely to be realised. If the mind is agitated, it will continue to be driven by fear, insecurity, attachment and desire, and will find it difficult to stay present and mindful. Most importantly, I learnt to challenge my thinking – to see that my thoughts could be functional but held little validity beyond that. Our thoughts and emotions are always changing, so how real can they be?

I downsized my life and cut out TV and newspapers. The effects of these teachings meant I no longer struggled or railed against things that happened – I became less likely to resist what life delivered to me in each moment, and understood the logic of accepting whatever happened. Vedanta gave me the confidence to understand that I was indeed whole and complete and that I didn't need material possessions or relationships to add anything to me or to make me happy. It's not that I didn't engage with these things – they were appreciated when I did – but I understood them for what they are. They were not providing me with lasting happiness, and therefore I didn't need to be attached to anything too much. I saw that I *was* the happiness; part of a divine whole and not separate from anything. Sometimes my mind still told me otherwise, however, and took me away from this. Toward the middle of 2011, I became very busy working and studying. Contemplation was put to one side, and that small voice of ignorance which would point out that I wasn't OK gnawed away at me.

Now I come to the real lesson Life had to teach me – something that couldn't be taught from a book. I was to be given a very difficult test. My worst fear had to be faced. At the beginning of 2011, when I was in India again, I was briefly hospitalised with an episode of dysentery, but seemed to be fine afterwards and continued to teach when I came back to the UK, running more courses. But in August of that year I was struck down with a mysterious fatigue-type illness. In many ways this mimicked the symptoms of ME that I had suffered from years before. My first reaction was one of terror – it was so frightening to experience something that I thought would never happen again, the complete and utter loss of all my energy. It felt as if my wiring had been pulled out. Initially I was too weak to leave the house and couldn't cook or shop for myself. Additionally I had severe muscle pains around my eyes which seemed to torture me day and night. This went on for weeks and I had to cancel more and more work. I had just started teaching philosophy on the Yoga Therapy Diploma course for Yoga Campus and was very sad when I realised that I would have to let that go. I gave up my yoga therapy work too, for the time being. I wasn't sure how I would survive financially and went to stay first with my friend Geri, then with my mother. But this time things were very different from when I was ill before. I now had many more tools to work with and this was the opportunity to put into practice what I had learnt over the past seven years, and what I had been teaching to my yoga students. In other words, I had to walk the walk and not just talk the talk. I needed to actually live the teachings from my heart and not just as something theoretical.

As a consequence of studying Vedanta and Yoga, I had been doing lots of self-inquiry; really looking into the fundamental nature behind the habits and identities that seemed to make up my personality. I could see that I had repeated a pattern, and had got caught up again in taking on too much work and making myself too busy which, ironically, was in opposition to the quiet and mindful yogic life I was teaching. I began to search myself; *why did I do this? Who was I really – prior to the thinking and behaviour?* It wasn't enough just to see the pattern, I needed to find what had caused it, or it would catch me out again, as our habits are hard-wired. I could see that my body, through its weakness and pain, was asking me to pay attention, to become more present and still. Indeed, I was too ill to do anything but be quiet and meditate.

My Vedanta teacher, who was now in America, emailed me a reminder that I keep with me to this day, "Take all action", he said, "only with peace as the goal. *You do not have to achieve anything. You do not have to please anyone. You do not have to be liked. You do not need to help anyone. You do not have to be successful and you do not need to be secure*". I printed this out in large, bold capitals. James was making the point that I needed to attend to myself before I could help others, and even then any action should only ever be from the heart - not from a need to please or for attention or to cover up insecurity. He was reminding me that I was actually fine, the real me was not touched by any of this. Later, James and I parted company for personal reasons but I will always be grateful for what he taught me during the time I was with him. He knew that, like many of us with a history of CFS, I had the pattern of being a people pleaser because I was still driven by the feeling of being separate and alone. This was largely unconscious, but had led me to take on too much work to prove to myself and the world that I was OK. I was coming from a place of fear and was chasing security outside of myself, and was very busy helping others whilst ignoring my own needs. I thought I had conquered these pattern years before, but evidently I hadn't, which just made it more insidious because it caught me off-guard. The ego (by which I mean the various identifications we take which drive our behaviour) is subtle - we think we have it under control but it slips back in with destructive behaviour when we least expect it. Unless we are prepared to really look deep inside and examine our unconscious thoughts and feelings and stay present with the dark stuff like depression, pain, insecurity and agitation, it will continue to trip us up. Now was the time to crack this. Nothing could be hidden anymore.

It was difficult., it took courage and vigilance. I realised how attached I was to being physically healthy, to travelling, socialising and working. This had all slipped from my grasp again - I was too ill to do much. There was a great deal of fear, but I also knew I had to accept and embrace what was happening and not wish for anything to be different - indeed how can we wish for anything to be other than it is? Resistance to what Is, and the thought that life shouldn't be exactly as it unfolds in each moment, is the basis of suffering. It really is that simple. I had to forgive myself too, for getting ill - for allowing this pattern to manifest itself again. I was greatly helped by my friend Alex Howard (of the Optimum Health Clinic) who coached me on the phone whenever I lost heart or had moments of despair. Sometimes I felt that I was unravelling, but Alex, who is a psychological therapist, has a great gift for pointing out the positive and reminded me that, although this was a steep learning curve, one day I would see it as a blessing and use it in my own teaching. He showed me that it really was different this time and that it was unhelpful to even think about when I had ME all those years ago. The memory is a trickster and can tell us something is going on when it actually isn't. Memory doesn't reference the truth from the stillness of now – it is just part of the mind which is always thinking about the past or the future. It is not real. Alex worked with love and from his heart.

Others supported me during this crisis, including my yoga mentor Gill Lloyd and my dear friends Leah Barnett, Ruth Heatherly, Geri Hollingworth, Jayne Roscoe, Martina Dodder, Liz Edwards, Katrina Heather and my mother. Gill gave me mantras around peace (*santih*) to work with. Julia Matschung, another friend, led by example, as she embodies and lives the teachings. She thoughtfully answered all my questions on the nature of suffering and self-realisation via email from Germany. These friends formed a circle of love around me and supported me as I struggled through. Karen Edwards, who is a self-realised teacher and who has health challenges herself, was a great inspiration to me. Through direct experience, she helped to show me the importance of listening to the truth of my heart – the authentic place of complete stillness that is always there, behind the noise of the mind.

During this time I had moments of great insight – and moments of great despair. I continued to be quiet and still and to observe what came up. I didn't use the label ME or Chronic Fatigue Syndrome, as to me those terms held negative connotations with what had been in the recent past and what was falsely anticipated in the future, which took away more vitality. The very words held a vibration that I didn't wish to engage in. It wasn't about denial, I just lived from moment to moment because that was all that really existed – anything else was only a false concept held in the mind. Sometimes there was energy, at others there was pain and profound fatigue. I learnt to accept; to not resist the symptoms and, more importantly, to not push away the *fear* of the symptoms when they came, but rather to welcome and nourish everything with compassion. I learnt to embrace my darker emotions and not to run away from them. I was brutally honest with myself and it was painful. Most of us push aside our bad feelings or try to medicate them with alcohol, TV, work, activity or other distractions. When we do this, energy is blocked as the emotion can't flow. Everything is energy – or *prana*. *Prana* needs to be able to move freely at all levels for true wellbeing, but it becomes trapped when we deny or turn away from our feelings – when we are not living authentically. Unconscious behaviour is often the result, which then causes us and others around us more suffering, fear and illness. The point was to bring all that was unseen to the light – something that I am still working on. I knew that I couldn't avoid anything now – the only way out of this was through it. Fear is always about the future, so this gave me an amazing opportunity to be present. When anxiety did creep in, I would see that it was just a thought and would come back to 'now' – to presence. It wasn't easy, especially when there was pain, but I just did what I could in each moment and tried to accept everything that arose or, if I couldn't, then to accept that I couldn't accept and that I was struggling! Sometimes the symptoms were very alarming. At times the fatigue was all-encompassing in a way which was, in itself, painful. My exhausted mind would drift into panic about the future and how I would survive. I watched the resistance. Yoga helped me to trust. There is a Sanskrit word we use from the Yoga Sutras: *Sraddha*. It means 'Faith and Trust'. Two books also helped me greatly, *'Falling Into Grace'* by Adyashanti (Sounds True publications) and *'The Presence Process'* by Michael Brown (Namaste Publishing). I thoroughly recommend them.

Meanwhile, I finally received a diagnosis of a parasite which had multiplied all over my system since the dysentery episode in India, so in May 2012, with the help of Charlotte Watts, a nutritionist and friend, I started on an anti-parasite herb. This initially exacerbated my symptoms and for a while I wasn't sure I was doing the right thing or taking the right medicine. For the time being, I had to continue to cancel much of my teaching, which reminded me of the karma yoga lesson – I, the individual, was not in control here. Something greater than me was, so I needed to let go and be grateful as each moment arose. I even questioned my identity as a yoga teacher and realised that it was possible I might end up 'doing' something else and that it was also possible to be too attached to yoga, Vedanta, meditation or even to the idea of being a 'spiritual' person. My identities were falling away to nothing. Whilst I was recovering, I watched Conscious TV on the internet (www.conscious.tv) and found many of the interviews very helpful, particularly one with the Advaita teacher Adyashanti, which I would urge anyone with CFS to watch. I also found the Byron Katie interview inspiring. Both told stories of suffering and sickness which had led them to freedom.

By August 2012 I had recovered. Again, like the first time I had been ill, I was very grateful for the lesson of being unwell – I could see that it was Grace and that it needed to happen for me to be forced to become still enough. This meant that I could finally understand, through contemplation, what I really needed to; the unhelpful patterns that

I needed to see through. My life is different now because of this experience; this lost year, which wasn't about loss at all – although in other ways it was about complete loss. My mind is much quieter; I enjoy spending more time alone in contemplation, I am open to what manifests in each moment and I have developed an inner stillness which feels very solid. I know everything comes and goes immediately, so there is no point holding on or being too attached to either the past or plans for the future. My insecurity, which I have faced up to and which I can see comes from the basic fear that we all have of feeling separate and alone, is dropping away and therefore any ambition I had has disappeared, which is the most tremendous relief. I have no need to achieve anything and nothing to prove to anyone any more, least of all myself. I no longer strive for anything or need attention. I know I am OK whatever happens. 'Let Go' is my mantra. To paraphrase Adyashanti: 'Life will give you what you need, and if you don't learn the lesson the first time it will keep being repeated until you do'.

I can now see that ill health comes from the many unconscious habits that we have and which we keep repeating. Illness is a way of making us pay attention. Until we really get to the bottom of what these patterns are, sickness may reoccur to remind us to stop, listen and learn. Making a drama out of illness and rushing around looking for a cure is not the answer – this is trying to find solutions in the mind rather than the heart. Real health comes from true peace. In fact, the idea of health is just a thought – a concept. So the most important lesson from all this for me was to learn to trust my own heart. I had another pattern to see through in order to appreciate this, that of putting teachers on pedestals in a way which disempowered me. But teachers – and scripture or, indeed, any teachings – can only take us so far. Ultimately we need to listen to our inner voice and to turn to that inner-nothingness, which is actually everything. Some traditions call this the Heart. No one else can do this for us.

I now see that wellness is a place of happiness, peace and acceptance right now, whatever the physical state of being. It is about the internal journey, or the identification of the one who is ever-present and unchanging, rather than the identity with states of health, which come and go. 'I am a sick person,' for example, brings in a whole story about illness yesterday and tomorrow and adds a huge burden to the mind. It is easier to change the internal environment (how we see things) rather than trying to manipulate the world around us, which includes our state of physical well-being. Someone or something may cause us pain, but we are responsible for what we then do with that thought and how we hold on to that. In other words, we are responsible for our own emotional reactions to everything, however bad. This is completely empowering, as it follows that we are actually in charge of our own suffering – it is a choice. So many times I have seen people with ME clutch on to the identity of being ill and of being a victim. Many are incredibly angry – with doctors, with society or even with their own families. The anger comes from fear – they are usually very frightened of the symptoms and will do anything to push them away, rather than staying present with them. Additionally, people with ME are often very driven and as soon as they have any energy they will start again on the ceaseless round of 'doing' and achieving, which just makes them ill again. The cure is to really face up to unconscious behavior from the root and to neutralise it by seeing what is really going on. Illness may bring about major life changes, including loss of income, status, relationship, home and social life. The tendency is to grasp at all of these with panic, but this will only bring about more suffering. If we can learn to fully let go, relax and trust what life is trying to show us, then we can use suffering as an opportunity to become still and peaceful; to practice deep self-inquiry and understand who we really are.

Many of the ideas from Vedanta and the philosophy from the Yoga Sutras, together with what I have studied as a KHYF teacher and, most importantly, what I have learnt from working with over 800 people with CFS over the last five years, are explored on my retreats. People usually come to yoga expecting a series of postures that will make them healthy, but it is actually a beautiful philosophy of balance, healing and wellbeing through empowerment – about understanding how to be happy with whom you really are in whatever situation you find yourself in. So, although yoga will certainly give you energy and vitality if you do some of the postures, it has so much more to offer. Ultimately it is about how to be peaceful, free and complete.

When I wrote the original book I didn't understand this myself as I hadn't yet studied at this level – and I wouldn't have been ready even if I had. I thought yoga was about a quiet mind and meditation – which it is to some degree – but this is just the foundation. The mind needs to be still enough before freedom can be understood. This may be realised through the process of discrimination between what is real (that which doesn't change – the Self) and what is always changing (everything else, including the body, mind and emotions). This is what real health is – being fully integrated on all levels of being. Ultimately yoga is really about unlinking from our identification to suffering (our life story) by the understanding of who we really are. People with chronic health challenges have an amazing opportunity, through their difficulties, to realise this.

I am now spending a lot of time in Spain writing. I have two book projects that I am working on. One is on yoga philosophy for healing and energy and the other is called '*The Guru in the Spare Room*' which about my time with a self-realised teacher, the student-teacher relationship, illness and the process of enlightenment. I write only for the joy of creation. I still run regular yoga retreats in the UK and abroad suitable for all abilities (www.fionaagombar.co.uk) and I hold teacher-training programmes on ME/CFS and Burnout for yoga teachers and health professionals through Yoga Campus and the British Wheel of Yoga. These courses are expanding all the time because CFS is sadly, a growing problem.

Other teachers such as Leah Barnett and Katrina Heather are now coming onboard, helping to raise standards, and we're beginning to receive interest in the course from outside the UK because yoga offers such an amazing tool box for self-healing for all chronic conditions – I call this the magic of yoga. I now teach in a way that, whilst embracing everything from the KHYF tradition, focuses on putting participants back in touch with their physical being and directs them to become present and quiet and therefore in touch with the authentic self. I teach like this because I understand the problem – I was out of touch with my own being for many years. Most people with CFS are usually very hyper-aroused and have an over-active, busy mind. This means that they are detached from the presence of who they are – and also from the body – so relaxation, letting go, staying present and non-judgemental and connecting with the physical being is a vitally starting point. I'm also interested in understanding how trauma can be released at the physical level, so this is something I also work with. I teach yoga as something creative, from my heart, so that whatever arises in each moment for me and the people I'm with is responded to in a way which brings about the maximum opportunity for healing – from the point of stillness. Until we learn to slow down and live mindfully in the flow of life and, rather than going against it by looking to the material for our peace, then I believe CFS, burnout and other conditions triggered by stress will continue to manifest themselves. Sadly, many people are uncomfortable about being quiet and will do anything to avoid this. Whilst we have continual cues from the environment telling us we're not good enough; that we need to buy more to be better, that we need the status of the right relationship or job and that we should be judged by what we have rather than by who we are, then we will continue to mistakenly and frantically rush around and reach outside ourselves for solutions, when the answer is that it is really an Inside job.

So for the time being I continue to write and teach and, best of all, meet lots of wonderful people. Most of all I like being still, marvelling at the wonder of life, however it manifest, and I hope that yoga can lead you to this inner joy too.

Fiona Agombar, August 2012

alex's story

by Alex Howard

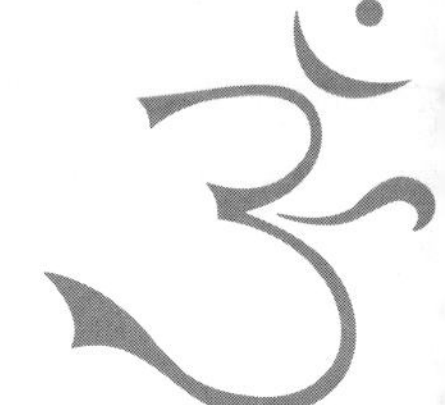

Up until the age of sixteen I was in many ways like most teenagers. I lived for three things: music, sport, and the opposite sex. School and homework were just something that had to be done to free up my time to embark upon these three passions. Like everyone I had heard about illnesses such as ME and CFS, but the idea of something like that happening to me was not even something I would have dreamed of. Spending seven years suffering from a severely debilitating chronic illness was about as likely as being on the next space shuttle to the moon and back.

Towards the end of my GCSEs I started to become tired and ended up in bed with a bad virus, but this was hardly surprising, and as far as I, the doctor, and my family were concerned, I just needed to rest for a while and I would be able to get back to enjoying the summer as usual. Ignorance really is bliss.

Three months later only really one thing had changed, I had another three months of practice for an uncertain, and at times almost unbearable, future under my belt. Tired of being unable to do anything, I made a desperate attempt to start at Sixth Form. Willpower got me through about ten days, before almost collapsing and spending weeks in bed just getting to the point that I could leave the house for a few minutes again. Struggling to get from the bedroom to the bathroom and back, and fit in a small amount of schoolwork became my daily struggle for the next two years. I quickly lost contact with my girlfriend, my friends, my hobbies, and in many ways the person I took to be myself.

After two years of living hell I reached the point that I simply couldn't take anymore. I'd already made major changes in my nutrition, which had included eating no sugar, yeast, wheat, preservatives or flavourings for the past two years. I had been to see numerous health practitioners, both conventional and otherwise, and still nothing had really changed. Depression was certainly not the cause of my miserable existence, but it was undoubtedly an inevitable consequence. As far as I was concerned it was looking like my life was over.

Just as I reached rock bottom, I called my uncle to tell him how I felt, in essence that I hated my life and everything about it. His response was very different to the typical response you might get in this situation. Rather than giving me sympathy or telling me that it would all be all right, he offered me something far more important. He asked me a series of life changing questions. The first of which was, "On a scale of 0-10, how badly do you want things to change?" After thinking about this for a few moments, I came to the conclusion that I was probably a 9 out of ten, I would do virtually anything to change my situation.

My uncle then asked me to make a list of all the things I thought I could do to change my situation, to which I added things like learning more about nutrition, practicing meditation and yoga on a consistent basis, learning how to get my mind into the right state to support my healing, and learning more about complementary health. He then asked me to list all the things that I felt made me worse. I had only one thing on this list: life. Just getting through the day felt like a major struggle on a daily basis.

After spending some time discussing these ideas, my uncle asked me a question that really made me think. The question was, "How many hours a day do you spend doing the things you yourself believe could make a difference?" The answer to this question was virtually none. So here I was, I wanted my life to change more than virtually anything, I had a rough idea of things I could do to change my situation, but I was consistently doing virtually nothing about it.

My uncle then asked me how many hours a day I spent watching television. The answer was about seven. Television had become my friend, it was the one thing that I could do that didn't require any real physical energy, and it meant that I could go off into another world and ignore the reality of my life. At the age of eighteen years old I had virtually a PhD in soap operas. This was hardly the vision I had had for my life. Looking around me I realised I wasn't the only person that was approaching their life with such a gaping difference between what I was saying I wanted, and what I was actually spending my life doing, but I also realised that most people in my situation don't recover, and I therefore couldn't afford to be like most people.

Over the next hour or so, my uncle helped me come up with a daily plan of how I could start to integrate my list of potentially helpful strategies into my daily routine. The commitments that I made included never watching more than two hours of television a day, doing thirty minutes meditation a day, five minutes yoga, starting to consistently read books on health and psychology, finding a meditation teacher, and to find a therapist to help look at my psychology.

For me at this point, I was too ill to sit in a chair and meditate for thirty minutes, so I would lie in a garden recliner kept in my bedroom to do so. My five minutes of yoga was really just doing yoga breathing, as I felt too weak to do any postures. However, I did have one essential resource; I was so desperate that I approached my commitments like my life depended upon them. I guess in many ways it did.

I soon realised that one of the things I needed were positive role models; essentially, people that had been through similar experiences to mine and found a way out, as the negativity around ME was becoming all-consuming. Struggling to find stories of people who had recovered from ME, I went in search of people who had recovered from other serious conditions. One story I came across had a particularly powerful impact upon me, this was the story of Meir Schneider. Meir was born blind, and after a number of failed operations in his early years, he was told there was no way he would ever be able to see. In his teenage years, Meir decided there was a whole world that he was missing out on, and that he would therefore do everything he could to find a way to see. Of course people around him thought he was either in denial or delusional, but Meir had a strength of spirit far beyond your average teenager.

One of the techniques that Meir came across was a technique called palming, which effectively involves staring at the sun with closed eyes, and slowly covering and uncovering your closed eyes with your hands. How many minutes in the average day do you think you could do this for before you became really, really, bored? Five minutes? Fifteen minutes? Meir used to do this technique for five hours a day, every single day. His level of commitment and resilience was in a league of its own.

Several years later, through this, and a number of other techniques, Meir's eyesight was virtually normal. Meir's story taught me something fundamental: If I was willing to give everything I could to my recovery, even though I could not yet see how it was possible, with persistence and perseverance perhaps I would find a way.

After six months of my new plan, and only marginal improvements, a new challenge unfolded for me: school. I was three months away from my A-levels, and having spent three years studying for them, I was still massively behind. The problem was that I needed A-levels to get to university, which to me seemed like the perfect answer. I mean what do students do all day? They sleep! Finally I was going to find somewhere that I would fit in! Secondly, students get student loans, and that was going to mean £15,000 to spend on my health.

At the school I attempted to attend, there was this joke about 'The Myth of Alex Howard' because I was hardly ever seen there. On one of the few afternoons I had been able to make it to class, the deputy headmaster spotted me walking through the schoolyard, and took what was a rare opportunity to have a word with me. He told me that considering how far behind I was, he felt it probably wasn't worth me continuing.

As part of what I had been reading to attempt to turn my health around, I had read a lot about the power of the mind to focus on something and make the impossible happen. Considering it was taking some time to turn my health around, I figured that perhaps this might be a good opportunity to test out this idea. The goal I set was to get straight As in my A-levels, something that virtually no-one achieves, especially considering my subjects were History, Economics and Business Studies, by no means easy options.

I spent the three months prior to my exams doing everything I could to teach myself all that I had missed. I only had about three hours a day that I was able to work for, so in these three hours I had to be totally focused, and I found that a number of accelerated learning techniques also made a big difference. Over these three months I taught myself a huge amount of work, and I caught up considerably. Unfortunately I pushed myself too hard. A week before my exams I had a major relapse.

I did end up taking my exams, but it took me four hours to do each three-hour exam. I would write my first essay over the allowed forty-five minutes. I would then lie in the bed next to my desk (I was taking my exams in the school's sick room) for twenty minutes until I was awoken by my supervisor. Then I would write an essay for another forty-five minutes. I would then sleep for twenty minutes. I would then write for forty-five minutes, sleep for another twenty minutes, and finally finish the exam. This was a rather painstaking way of doing it, but even this was an incredible strain on me, and to this day I have very little recollection of this whole period.

When I got my A-level results I got a very rude awakening. A rude awakening to the true power of the human spirit. I had achieved my goal. I got straight As, along with the highest marks in the school in some of my papers. This greatly strengthened my resolve, and I got back to working intensely on turning around my health for another three years.

These three years at university were the period where I really went on my journey with true conviction. Every minute I was awake was about understanding my health and self. I read over five hundred books on all different kinds of psychology, spirituality, energy work, hypnosis, meditation, health, and anything else that might hold the answers to my inner journey. Much of the time was incredibly lonely, for there was often no one that I could share my experiences or journey with. Yet, something else that I learnt is that it is in the deepest loneliness and pain that we hear the most important voice of all: the voice of our soul and spirit, and it was this that I constantly aligned myself with.

There were times when I read a passage in a book that would touch me on a profound level, and because I had no one to share it with, in some ways it touched me even more deeply. I spent countless hours in meditation and practicing yoga, and as my health slowly returned I started to go for longer and longer walks along Swansea Bay, dragging my frail body with unstoppable determination a few steps further each time.

Towards the end of my first year at university, my uncle invited me to go along to a yoga weekend with Simon Lowe. It was a major turning point for me. Prior to the weekend I had been extremely nervous that I would be able to do four yoga classes in a couple of days, as at this point I had never even been to a full class before. By really learning to listen to my body, I discovered that in a calm and centred state I was able to do more than at that time I had believed I could do.

At the weekend I also met Sue Delf (who teaches on the DVD which accompanies this book, along with Fiona Agombar), and for the summer break following I went to several of her classes each week. Once I got back to University I continued with my yoga practice and was eventually doing around forty-five minutes every day. It felt incredible to be able to build up from primarily doing breathing exercises and gentle postures to being able to do what eventually became a real workout.

At the end of these three years I earned a first class degree in psychology (for which I had won the Best Student Award from the British Psychological Society), as well as getting an advanced diploma in clinical hypnotherapy, neuro-linguistic programming and life coaching (I did my post-graduate training at the same time as the third year of my degree – quadrupling my reading speed had made studying a lot easier). Far more important than this was the fact that I had been able to take great strides forward in my health. Upon leaving university I went into practice with my teacher in hypnotherapy and moved to London. It seemed that the more I learnt about human psychology, the more changes I was able to make in my life.

Another six months later, and I had made a full recovery. Like most people who are seriously ill, I had a benchmark that once I reached I knew I had made it. For me this was to be able to go for a run with no ill effects afterwards. This was something I had dreamt about doing for seven years, and to say it was an amazing feeling is perhaps the greatest understatement possible.

In the three years since then, a whole new journey has opened up and unfolded. With the publication of my auto-biographical story *WHY ME? My Journey From ME To Health And Happiness*, and the results I was starting to get in the clinic working with other sufferers, I soon found myself inundated with people seeking help on their own healing journeys. I quickly brought on board a clinical nutritionist, and the clinic since then has grown from strength to strength. In time the clinic moved to Harley Street, and yet we still found a way of keeping our prices affordable and our level of personal support and customer service second to none.

We essentially take the approach that everyone's body is different, and therefore helping each person requires a whole investigative process in of itself. Yet what we have also found is that there are clear commonalities, and having treated hundreds of people ranging from those that are totally bedbound and living in darkened and sound proofed rooms due to extreme light and sound sensitivities, to people who are burnt out but still able to work as undercover policeman, I can honestly say that it is possible for everyone with fatigue to significantly improve their situation.

We have seen results as dramatic as people who are wheelchair bound and suicidal due to extreme fatigue fully recover in as little as three months. If you'd like to discover more about our approach, you can download a free e-book and you can order a free CD on our treatments with ME at www.TheOptimumHealthClinic.com

For me personally, yoga is one of the many gifts that my illness has brought me. I still practice on a very regular basis, and yoga is one of my favourite ways of connecting with myself. We have also found Fiona's book to be of great value to patients at the clinic, as it helps people find a way to very slowly and gently get their body moving (once their physical energy has started to increase) and reap the numerous benefits that yoga has to offer.

I guess the most important lesson from my own journey was that we often take so many things in life for granted, and when we lose something as fundamental as our energy we are forced to look at and consider what in our life really matters. Perhaps this is the real reason why so many people in our modern world are struggling with the energy, and yoga is a great way to embark upon or accelerate this journey of understanding.

If you'd like to order a copy of Alex Howard's first book, *WHY ME? My Journey From ME To Health And Happiness*, please also visit www.TheOptimumHealthClinic.com

15 alex's postscript

October 2012

It seems that so much has happened in both my life (and Fiona's!) since I wrote a shortened version of my story to be included in her book. As far as my personal life is concerned, I got married, had a daughter, and continue to enjoy the passion for life that was born out of the years I was so desperately ill. Of course, with each year of life comes new lessons and new adventures, but one thing you can be sure of is that as the journey never ends, and neither does our potential for appreciation and gratitude for that journey.

With regard to the treatment and understanding of fatigue, and more specifically chronic fatigue and ME, I think we are in very exciting times. The complex interaction between mind and body is becoming clearer, the physical imbalances that also play an important role are increasingly well understood, and new approaches are being evolved all the time to tackle these areas. With the development of resources such as the internet, it has become so much easier to find inspiration, connect with others on a similar journey, and to hopefully find the answers we are searching for. We still have a way to go, but progress is most definitely being made.

Although I know that dealing with health issues can be very challenging, I think it's immensely important that people understand that there are answers out there. Everybody is obviously different, and yet there are clear patterns. Having supervised the treatment of thousands of people with ME/CFS in over thirty five countries around the world through my work with The Optimum Health Clinic, I can honestly say that whatever the situation, it is almost always possible to improve it. It's one thing for me to know that, another for the patient to begin to believe it, and I think a great step towards supporting that belief is connecting with the stories of others that have been down the same path. It's a path which seems to be becoming increasingly well-trodden.

Best wishes on your journey to optimum health!

summary

Here's a reminder of the main points of this book – the things you might like to try to Beat Fatigue with Yoga!

- Firstly, be aware of your health. Start to tune in to how you feel every day and what makes you feel well.
- Practise some yoga postures regularly – especially the Pose of Complete Rest.
- Take enough rest and relaxation and make time for yourself.
- Check your posture regularly.
- Eat as nutritious a diet as you can.
- Drink lots of water.
- Practise breathing slowly and rhythmically using your diaphragm.
- Try using some of the special yoga breathing exercises from Chapter 4.
- Sit outside in the fresh air and sunshine, visit the seaside or the mountains, and walk barefoot to take in extra prana whenever possible.
- Avoid pollution, dust and smoke as these zap vital energy.
- Meditate for 10-20 minutes every day.
- Take responsibility for your own health – some of us treat our cars better than our bodies! Respect yourself and your health.
- Remember, positive thinking raises prana, so try and see the good things in your life and don't focus on the bad things.
- Try to live in the present moment and keep your mind calm.

Good Luck!

glossary

Prana	Universal life energy
Asana	Yoga posture
Pranayama	Yoga breathing
Chakra	Energy centre in the body
Nadi	Channel for vital energy
Mantra	A word, phrase or sound which has meaning
Bandha	A position used to lock in energy
Mudra	A hand position to direct energy flow

bibliography

Ajaya, Swami, *Yoga Psychology*, The Himalayan lnternational Institute of Yoga Science and philosophy, 1976

Bell, Lorna, and Seyfer, Eudora, *Gentle Yoga*, Celestial Arts, 1982

Brennan, Barbara, *Hands of Light*, Bantam, 1987

Brennan, Barbara, *Light Emerging*, Bantam, 1993

Capra, Fritjof, *The Tao of Physics*, Flamingo, 1982

Carter, Jill, and Edwards, Alison, *The Elimination Diet Cookbook*, Element Books, 1997

Carter, Jill, and Edwards, Alison, *The Rotation Diet Cookbook*, Element Books, 1997

Chaitow, Leon, *The Beat Fatigue Workbook*, Thorsons, 1988

Crawford, Moira, *The Natural Way with Allergies*, Element Books, 1997

Devereux, Godfrey, *The Elements of Yoga*, Element Books, 1994

Eastcott, Michal, *The Silent Path*, Rider, 1989

Freedman, Miriam, and Hankes, Janice, *Yoga at Work*, Element Books, 1996

Heilbronn, Bill, *The Yoga Students' Companion*, published by the author, 1995

Isaacson, Cheryl, *Thorsons Principles of Yoga*, Thorsons, 1996

Iyengar, B.S.K., *Light on Yoga*, Thorsons, 1991

Jacobs, Gill, *The Natural Way: Chronic Fatigue Syndrome*, Element Books, 1997

Jacobs, Gill, and Kjaer, Joanna, *Beat Candida Through Diet*, Vermillion, 1997

Kelder, Peter, *Tibetan Secrets of Youth and Vitality*, Thorsons, 1988

Kent, Howard, *Breathe Better; Feel Better*, Apple Press, 1997

Kent, Howard, *The Complete Yoga Course*, Headline, 1995

Martin, Simon, *The Natural Way with Candida*, Element Books, 1998

Mehta, Silva, Mira and Shyam, *Yoga the Iyengar Way*, Dorling Kindersley, 1995
Muktananda, Swami, *Where are you Going?*, Gurudev Siddha Peeth, 1982
Nagarathna, Dr P., Nagendra, Dr H.R., and Monro, Dr P., *Yoga for Common Ailments*, Gaia Books, 1990
Ozaniec, Naomi, *The Elements of the Chakras*, Element Books, 1996
Page, Dr Christine, *Frontiers of Health*, The C.W. Daniel Company Ltd, 1996
Purna, Dr Svami, *Yoga, a Practical Introduction*, Element Books, 1998
Ramacharaka, Yogi, *The Hindu Yogi Science of Breath*, LAN. Fowler and Co. Ltd, 1960
Sears, Barry, *Enter the Zone*, Regan Books, 1995
Sivananda, Swami, *The Science of Pranayama*, The Divine Life Society, 1992
Sivananda Yoga Centre, *The Book of Yoga*, Ebury Press, 1995
Smith, Erica, and Wilks, Nicholas, *Meditation*, Vermillion, 1997
Stewart, Dr Alan, *Tired All the Time*, Optima, 1993
Sturgess, Stephen, *The Yoga Book*, Element Books, 1997
Tobias, Maxine, and Stewart, Mary, *Stretch and Relax*, Dorling Kindersey, 1995
Van Lysebeth, Andre, *Pranayama*, Unwin, 1983
Vollmar V, *Journey Through the Chakras*, Gateway Books, 1992
White, Ruth, *Working with Your Chakras*, Piatkus, 1993
Yogananda, Sri Sri Paramhansa, *Autobiography of a Yogi*, Jaico Publishing House, 1975

Bibliography for the Second Edition

Dillman, E., *The Little Book of Yoga*, Warner Books, 1998
Ekhart Tolle, *The Power of Now*, Hodder and Stoughton 1999
Francis, Timothy C. *Patanjali's Steps of Yoga*, Wessex Aquarian, 1997
Howard, Alex, *Why ME? My Journey From ME To Health And Happiness*, Roximillion Publications, 2003
Jacobs, G., *Chronic Fatigue Syndrome*, Element Books, 1997
MacGregor, Jan, interview with Dr David Mason Brown, *Interaction*, June 2001, or visit www.cfs-me.com
Pheby, Dr D., 'Management and Treatment of ME', *Positive Health*, October 2000

Shepherd, Dr C., MB BS et al., *ME/CFS/PVFS An Exploration of the Key Clinical Issues*, The ME Association, 2001
Sieverling, C., *Dr Cheney's Basic Treatment Plan for CFS*, published on the Internet, details: lsieverl@flash.net
Wright, Dr A., MBChB DPCOG MPCGP DCH DiHom, *Chronic Fatigue Syndrome (ME)/Fibromyalgia and Associated Syndromes*, Chronobiology Ltd, 2001

Bibliography for the Third Edition

Adyashanti, *Falling Into Grace*, Sound True, 2011
Farhi, Donna, *Bringing Yoga to Life*, Harper One, 2003
Brown, Michael, *The Presence Process*, Namaste Publishing, 2010
Wilson, James L, ND. DC,PhD, *Adrenal Fatigue The 21st Century Stress Sundrome*, Smart Publications, 2000
Desikachar, TKV, *The Heart of Yoga*, Inner Traditions International, 1995
Adyshanti, *True Meditation*, Sounds True Publications 2006 (includes a wonderful free CD).
Tolle, Eckhart, *A New Earth*, Penguin 2005

useful addresses

Action for ME has a very good journal and membership service. Action for ME, 3rd Floor, Canningford House, 38 Victoria Street, Bristol, BS1 6BY www.afme.org.uk

Alex Howard runs a clinic to help support those with ME. He offers excellent advice on the best diet to gain optimum health and energy and also offers therapy services such as NLP. His book *Why ME? My Journey From ME To Health And Happiness* published by Roximllion Publications/Cherry Red books is also available from: the Optimum Health Clinic, 1-7 Harley Street, London W1G 9QD or contact: alex@theoptimumhealthclinic.com. The DVD, *Beat Fatigue with Yoga*, which includes a 25 minute session for people with ME, is also available from this address.

Angela Stevens has excellent cassette tapes with yoga for ME sessions on them. Angela also keeps a list of teachers across the UK who specialise in teaching yoga for ME so if you want to know if there is a teacher in your area send an SAE to: Angela Stevens, Laminga, Southview Road, Wadhurst, East Sussex, TN5 6TL.

Dr Andy Wright runs a clinic and offers lots of help on nutrition. Chronobiology, 57 Chorley New Road, Bolton, BL1 4QR or e mail: chronobiologyuk@yahoo.co.uk

Asquith make great clothes for doing yoga in – I used their bootcut trousers for this book. They also make really good comfortable clothes to relax in, so if you are feeling tired you can look smart and comfortable at the same time – without too much effort. www.asquith.ltd.uk or for a catalogue call 0208 968 3100.

Brainfog is an excellent online-support group for people with M.E. Run by Alison Petty, the site has won awards for its design and innovation. Brainfog also run gatherings. I sometimes take yoga retreats for Brainfog. Click www.Brainfog.org.

KHYF (Krishnamachary Healing and Yoga Foundation) offer courses and teacher training. More information from www.khyf.co.uk

The ME Association is also a good national charity for people with ME.
ME Association, 4, Top Angel, Buckingham Industrial Estate, Buckingham, MK18 1TH.
01280 816115

Revival is a holistic health and yoga centre in West London. All the products used are environmentally friendly – there are no chemicals in any of the treatments. (Although if you are chemically sensitive please note that oils and incense are used.) Massage, reiki, sacro-cranial therapy and homeopathy are just some of the treatments available and all the therapists are excellent. I run classes there three times a week. Revival, 227 High Road, Chiswick, London W4.

The Special Yoga Centre runs general and therapeutic classes including a weekly class for people with ME. The Special Yoga Centre has an amazing peaceful atmosphere, is run by true yogis and also offers classes for children with special needs. The Special Yoga Centre, 2a Wrentham Avenue, Kensal Rise NW10.
0208 968 1930

Tanya Roche. If you ever need a cheerful, helpful and professional photographer then contact Tanya on 07956 423521. www.tanyaroche.co.uk

Tim Francis has written an excellent interpretation of the sutras of Patanjali if you are interested in exploring yoga philosophy further. The book is available from the author at £4.00 which covers post and packing: Tim Francis, 8 Cave's Court, Potton, Bedfordshire, SG19 2PW.

I have a web site which gives regular updates of yoga classes and retreats and the DVD to go with this book. You can also contact me via my website:
www.fionaagombar.co.uk

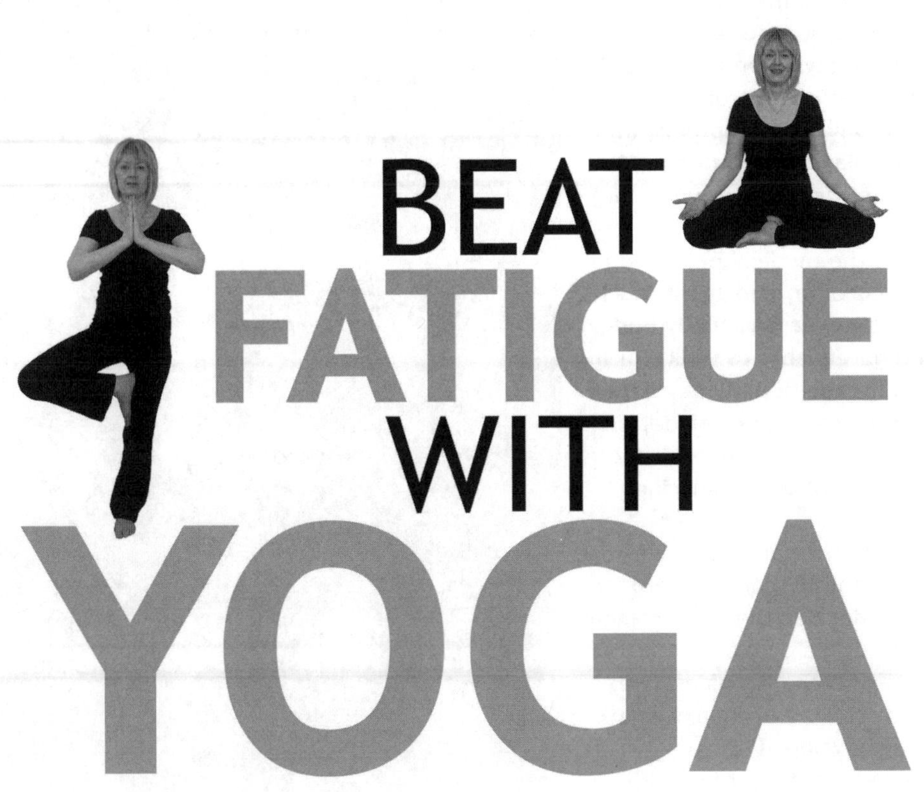

beat fatigue with yoga

The DVD with Fiona Agombar and Sue Delf

This DVD is the essential companion to this book. Contains three separate yoga classes for different levels of energy. Also interviews with Fiona Agombar, Sue Delf and Alex Howard